Curing the Cancer in U.S. Healthcare:

StatesCare and the Texas Model

Curing the Cancer in U.S. Healthcare:

StatesCare and the Texas Model

By
Dr. Deane Waldman, MD, MBA

Strategic Book Publishing and Rights Co.

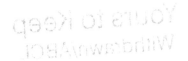

Dedication

This work is dedicated to all my fellow sufferers, those who choose to provide health care to others, and when needed, hospice relief. If you, dear reader, provide health care, you know much of what follows. You live it every day and carry on despite your suffering.

If you don't work in healthcare, let me paint you a picture, one that shows care providers in chains. They do what society and patients want. They assume, with good reason, that the system will help them do their good and noble work. U.S. healthcare does precisely the opposite.

Your doctor doesn't really practice medicine on you. An insurance actuary or government regulator tells the doctor what drug you can take, what operation you can have, how long you have to wait before you get the care you need, and if you get it, ever! Neither the doctor nor the patient is the medical decision maker.

Every day, virtually every U.S. physician will fight with an insurance bureaucrat to try to get you the care you need. All too often, the doctor will lose … and so will you.

Just like doctors, nurses are forced to waste hours each day on administrative tasks and regulatory compliance that do not help patients. Those hours spent in front of a computer screen are hours they can't be with their patients.

The system in which health care providers must function is designed to obstruct, restrain, control, penalize, and punish rather than help them as they struggle to help you.

This book honors all those who get up every morning knowing they will have to push back against the very system that should encourage, support, and reward them. Health care providers—nurses, doctors, and therapists of all kinds—do this out of dedication to patient welfare. This book is dedicated to them.

About the Author

Why should you read what Dr. Deane writes? Because he is your "go to" guy if you want to understand your healthcare system, and more importantly, know what to do about it. With both an MD and MBA, Dr. Deane is your most credible source for six reasons:

1. Education and training at Yale, Chicago Med, Mayo Clinic, Northwestern, Harvard, and Anderson Management School;
2. He is Director of the Center for Health Care Policy at the Texas Public Policy Foundation based in Austin, Texas;
3. During almost 40 years as a pediatric cardiologist, he has experienced every aspect of healthcare, including being a patient himself in an ICU, twice;
4. Dr. Deane is able to make our healthcare system understandable to the average person; and,
5. He has no political agenda. Dr. Deane simply wants to treat a sick system we call Patient Healthcare using the principles of good medical practice.

Dr. Deane is a widely recognized authority, both speaking as well as writing articles and books. He has published more than 140 academic medical articles and monographs along with more than 300 articles for the general public about healthcare. He is a contributor to *Huffington Post, American Thinker, The Blaze, The Hill, RealClearHealth, The Federalist, Investor's Business Daily,* and *The Washington Examiner,* as well as newspapers including *USA Today, Houston Chronicle,* and *The Wall Street Journal.* Dr. Deane is interviewed frequently on radio.

Dr. Deane has published four print books titled, *Uproot U.S. Healthcare, 2nd Edition; Cambio Radical al Sistema de Salud de los Estados Unidos* (Spanish translation of the *Uproot* book); multiple award-winner *The Cancer in Healthcare;* and award-winning *The Cancer in the American Healthcare System.* He has released six of the seven eBooks in the best-selling series, *Restoring Care to American Healthcare.*

Outside of medicine, Dr. Deane has had some … *interesting* life experiences. As a child, he was in the Middle East when the 1956 War broke out. He was an exchange student in Berlin in 1961 when the Wall went up between East and West Germany. Thirty-seven years later in 1998, Dr. Deane had the pleasure of revisiting Berlin, with the Wall gone and the city reunited. In 1968, Dr. Deane patched up the injured during the Democratic National Convention in Chicago, and in 2013, he acted as "war correspondent" writing articles for *The Blaze* from Istanbul during the Silent Revolution. Dr. Deane says his life priorities are: his family, We the Patients, and bicycling on the track (velodrome), in that order.

This book is a print version of eBook #6 from the series, *Restoring Care to American Healthcare,* with numerous updates and additional figures. It is also the logical conclusion to *The Cancer in the American Healthcare System,* which established the root cause for failure of our healthcare system. This book shows the cure.

Table of Contents

Introduction

To cure sickness, you need to know the cause, whether the patient is a sick human or a critically ill system like healthcare. Otherwise, you can only palliate the patient's symptoms rather than curing him, her or it.

The main symptoms in U.S. healthcare are apparent to everyone: too expensive and too little care. Costs are incredible, you can't find a doctor, and when you do find one, you have to wait four months to get an appointment.

Healthcare costs are eating our lunch, along with breakfast, dinner and the mortgage payment! Look at the facts in the summary below starting with the average American family of four based on a Milliman Medical Index and Income Survey from January 2018.[1] The family foregoes more than $13,000 of income in employer support for insurance premium expenses, and pays almost half of their take-home pay for out-of-pocket health costs.

Family Budget	Amount	Percentages
Take-home (gross) salary	$58,829	81%
Employer pays for your insurance premiums	$13,430	19%
Potential take-home salary	$72,259	100%
Family healthcare costs		

Co-pays and deductible (out-of-pocket)	$ 8,685	31%
Insurance premiums (out-of-pocket)	$ 6,050	21%
Employer-paid premiums	$13,430	48%
Total family annual healthcare costs	$28,165	100%
Healthcare costs as percentage of take-home pay		48%

Most American families simply cannot afford this. Yet, insurance costs keep rising despite the self-styled "Affordable" Care Act of 2010. The nation cannot afford healthcare either. In 1960, the U.S. expended 5 percent of Gross Domestic Product (GDP) on healthcare. In 2018, healthcare will consume more than 18 percent of GDP.

"Healthcare" as one word means the system, one that is overspending us into bankruptcy and incurring debt that our children will have to pay back. "Health" . . . "care" as two words is personal service provided by a professional, something that is harder and harder to get, especially in time to save us from illness and death.

Healthcare has been described as a "broken" system. I prefer to view our failing system as a sick person. As such, Patient Healthcare is in the ICU on life support.

While we agree how sick healthcare is, people disagree on what to do. Some say we should repeal and replace Obamacare, but sadly, they have no idea what the replacement should be. Some claim that single payer is the answer.[2] People speak with great passion but often have little evidence. Most Americans are simply confused and frustrated. They know both political parties make promises that fail to materialize. Americans know what they don't want but are unclear about what they do want.

Curing our failing healthcare system starts with knowing the cause of illness. I wrote *The Cancer in the American Healthcare System* in order to take readers through the thinking process doctors use when making an etiologic or causative diagnosis. Systems thinkers describe this activity as root cause analysis. In the previous book, we uncovered that the reason U.S. healthcare is failing both Americans and the nation: cancer.

Our healthcare system has cancer located in the federal bureaucracy. It keeps growing and growing apparently without limit, consuming healthcare funds that are desperately needed to pay for care. The book you hold starts with the diagnosis of cancer and goes from there. It shows how we can fix healthcare so that Americans can get the care they need, when and where they need it, at a price we can afford both as individuals and as a nation.

Chapter Notes

1. The 2018 Milliman Medical Index can be found at: www.milliman.com/mmi.
2. In a book titled, "Single Payer Won't Save Us," I collected all the evidence and results for single payer systems in Great Britain, Canada, and even our own homegrown single payer disaster, the VA system. *The title gives you what I think about single payer. However, you should decide for yourself, based on hard evidence not emotional rhetoric.*

Chapter 1:

Healthcare Is Critically Ill

You are a doctor. A patient walks into your office complaining of headaches. You introduce yourself and sit down in front of your computer. You find a pain killer that is authorized by the patient's health plan in its Pharmacy Benefits Management Program. You then print the prescription, using only a government-approved printer, of course. You hand the top copy of the triplicate form to the patient. The receptionist gives the patient a Bill for Services Rendered and ushers him out the door. You have successfully *cared for* the patient within your allotted 15-minute increment and will get high marks on your efficiency scorecard.

No history taken. No physical exam performed. No lab tests or imaging of any kind—MRI, X-ray, echo, or CT scan. No review of patient's medical records or reading of previous medical literature on other patients with similar complaints. No differential diagnosis. No attempt to find the cause of the patient's symptoms. Just a painkiller and out the door. Was this good medical practice? If you were this patient, would you be satisfied? Of course not!

That is precisely how Congress has *treated* a "patient" called the U.S. Healthcare System for more than five decades. Federal solutions invariably unfold the same way. They announce a crisis in healthcare, write new regulations, and thus spend more money on the federal bureaucracy, leaving fewer and fewer dollars to spend on care that patients need.

No wonder Patient Healthcare is now critically ill in the ICU on life support. Absent a miracle, Patient Healthcare is going to die. When that happens, Americans will no longer be able to get the lifesaving they need. Then, as some politicians have predicted, we will see people "dying needlessly in the streets."

Washington's fixes-that-fail-or-backfire

Medicare was created as part of the Social Security Act of 1965. It was supposed to be a giant, national savings account that would provide for our medical needs after retirement. The Congressional Budget Office (CBO) promised Congress the program would cost $12 billion. In fact, 25 years after passage, a financial audit of the Medicare program found that Congress underestimated the expense by an astonishing 854 percent! Instead of $12 billion, Medicare cost more than $100 billion.

The CBO now predicts the Medicare Trust Fund will be insolvent by 2026.[1] This means Medicare will be unable to pay for senior medical needs like drugs, nursing care, operations, etc. Those who contributed for forty years of work life and were promised medical security in retirement will be left out in the cold. Grandma will fall off the ledge because Medicare won't be able to pay for her walker, much less a wheelchair.

The year 1965 saw not only the creation of Medicare, but Medicaid as well, both parts of President Lyndon Johnson's Great Society. Medicaid was jointly funded by both the states and the federal government. The law provided for 51 distinctly different programs, each one administered by the individual state or the District of Columbia. Section 1801 in the 1965 Medicaid law confirmed that the states were supposed to be in charge of their own programs. The title was, "Prohibition against any federal interference."[2]

Slowly, piece by piece, rule by rule, Washington took over administration of every aspect of state Medicaid programs, implementing a federal, centralized, one-size-fits-all approach. [3] When I write "every aspect of state Medicaid programs, that is not hyperbole. When New Mexico was creating its Health Insurance Exchange, the Washington-based Centers for Medicare and Medicaid Services (CMS) even dictated the font (typeface) and type size of the eligibility forms that patients must complete.

One size does not fit all. It doesn't even fit most! Any single healthcare mandate does not apply equally to all Americans, in our diverse regions, with a wide variety of medical needs and different resources.

Medicaid has grown to be the largest single line item in most state budgets. Yet, the states do not control where this money goes—Washington does. As a result of Washington's takeover of administrative control over state Medicaid programs, they are failing both enrollees and our nation.

Entitlement reform is a favorite sound bite for both parties. Both Democrats and Republicans claim their party's latest fix will solve the Medicaid entitlement problem, yet they never really "fix" anything. The solution is always the same: more government, more regulations, more spending, and blaming the previous administration for the ever-growing entitlement monster.

Figure 1-1: A Bipartisan Approach to Medicaid

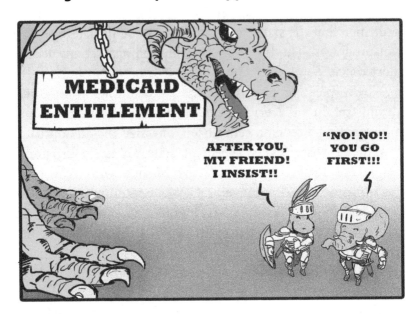

Systems theory[4] is the study of how systems such as organizations, institutions, and even government agencies function, particularly when they are failing. This discipline has a term that describes both Medicare and Medicaid: fixes-that-failed-or-backfired. This means there is a problem with the program, that a solution was implemented to fix the problem, and that the problem was not fixed or actually got worse.

Washington's fixes for Medicare "backfired" so that, in less than ten years, Medicare will leave seniors without medical care. The expansion of Medicaid pursuant to implementing Obamacare, caused state programs to "backfire" by reducing the availability of care for the people who need it most (Figure 1-2).

In the early twentieth century, people who needed medical care but could not pay for it received their care either through private charities or in county-supported hospitals.[5] With the collapse of the county hospital system in the 1960s, sick indigent persons and poor pregnant women began showing up in large numbers in hospital emergency rooms. Hospitals started playing a game of hot potato. They *dumped* critically ill, non-paying patients to other hospitals.

In the 1980s, newspapers started headlining tragedies like, "Mother Dies Giving Birth in Alley," and "If You're Sick and Poor, Too Bad." Without any hard evidence, Congress passed EMTALA (Emergency Medical Transport and Labor Act of 1985) also known as the "anti-dumping" law. EMTALA said that hospitals accepting federal funds, i.e., almost all U.S. hospitals, and having an emergency room, were required to "provide for an appropriate medical screening examination … [and] such treatment as may be required to stabilize the medical condition," whether the patient had insurance or not.[6] An uninsured person having a heart attack could enter the ER, be sent to the ICU, and receive all necessary care including open heart surgery, without having any payment source to cover the hospital bill.

EMTALA created a huge, federally mandated financial loss for hospitals. "Huge" is no exaggeration. The average profit margin for most large urban hospitals is roughly two percent. The cost of uncompensated care is typically at least 20 percent of a hospital's operating budget.[7] Hospitals were forced to adopt creative accounting tricks and shady billing practices, or otherwise they had to close their doors. By solving one problem—care for the uninsured—EMTALA created another one: the unfunded mandate.

The CEO of a well-known insurance company had a hernia repair at a famous hospital. (The CEO's name is withheld for his own protection.) At discharge, he was handed a bill for $28,440.28. Believing the cost was exorbitant, the insurance CEO went to talk with the hospital's Chief Financial Officer

Figure 1-2: Medicaid Expansion Reduces Access to Care

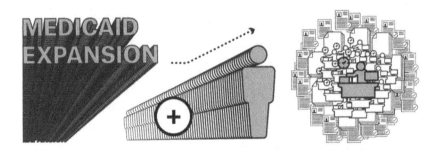

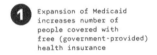

1 Expansion of Medicaid increases number of people covered with free (government-provided) health insurance

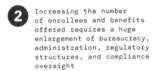

2 Increasing the number of enrollees and benefits offered requires a huge enlargement of bureaucracy, administration, regulatory structures, and compliance oversight

(CFO). Line by line, item by item, service by service, they went through the five-page bill. Each time, the CEO demurred saying the charge was too high. Finally, the CFO threw up his hands exclaiming, "Blame EMTALA, not me. The excessive charges on your bill pay for the care of people who have no insurance."

The Health Insurance Portability and Accountability Act of 1996 (HIPAA) was another example of a Washington fix-that-fails-or-backfires. In the mid-1990s, many people were losing their jobs. Most workers had employer-supported health insurance through their jobs. As companies had to reduce their operating costs, they used "reductions in force," or "RIFs," a nicer way of saying the company was getting rid of their employees. When people lost jobs, families lost employer-supported health insurance coverage. Congress said HIPAA would make health insurance portable across the job market.

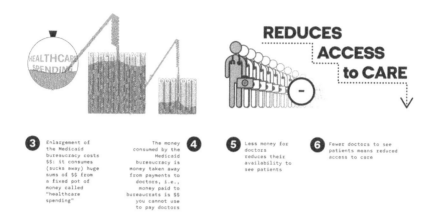

3 Enlargement of the Medicaid bureaucracy costs $$: it consumes (sucks away) huge sums of $$ from a fixed pot of money called "healthcare spending"

4 The money consumed by the Medicaid bureaucracy is money taken away from payments to doctors, i.e., money paid to bureaucrats is $$ you cannot use to pay doctors

5 Less money for doctors reduces their availability to see patients

6 Fewer doctors to see patients means reduced access to care

HIPAA failed to make insurance portable, certainly not in any affordable way. It did expand Medicaid eligibility, but how is that related to portability? By tightening the security protocols for sharing medical information, HIPAA made communication between care providers *much* more difficult. As a result, the likelihood of medical errors *increased*![8] HIPAA joins the group of Washington's fixes-that-fail-or-backfire.

Congress's most recent "fix" for our sick healthcare system is the Affordable Care Act (ACA). When you strip away all the political hyperbole and disinformation, the ACA has been proven to produce the following results:

1. Insurance has become more expensive, not less expensive.
2. Access to care has gone down--care has become less available.
3. Washington has spent an additional $1.8 trillion, bending the cost curve upward![9] (The GDP of Canada is $1.8 trillion.)

4. Many patients cannot keep the doctor they like, in contrast to what was promised.
5. Maneuvering the ACA website and structure to access government-approved insurance plans is nothing short of torture.[10]
6. If an ACA insurance plan is chosen, the forms (i.e., 1095-A, 8962) and tax ramifications for subsidies are additional nightmares for patients.

Washington's behavior is clear and repetitive. They identify a problem, call it a crisis, and use the so-called "impending disaster" as a lever to expand government administration and regulatory authority, and then spend more money on bureaucracy, taking it away from care.

Proof

There is a mountain of evidence showing bad medical outcomes in patients with government-supplied insurance. The fiscal impacts are equally negative, both for the individual and our country.

Is Our Care Sufficient to Our Needs?

A February 2017 national survey[11] reported that the maximum wait time to see a family physician in mid-sized U.S. cities had risen to 122 days. That is four months to find out if the pain in your belly is gas, an ulcer, or cancer.

An internal audit[12] of the Veterans Affairs (VA) health system concluded, "307,000 veterans may have died waiting for approval for medical care." Our military veterans experienced "death-by-queueing" just as Britons do in their vaunted NHS

(National Health Service) as well as our neighbors to the north in Canada.[13]

Death-by-queueing refers to a person dying from a treatable illness while waiting to get care that could have saved his life if it were provided in time. For example, burn victims are more likely to survive if cared for in specialized Burn Units rather than in a general hospital environment. Canada has allocated an amount of money for a number of Burn Units that is insufficient for the number of burn victims. There is a long waiting list to get in. People die waiting in line who might be saved if they could have been admitted to a Burn Unit.

There are numerous reports of government-insured Americans dying because they couldn't get needed care in time. Deamonte Driver was a 12-year-old Maryland boy who died from complications of a cavity in a tooth.[14] He couldn't get dental care because the Medicaid dental reimbursement schedules were too low, and there were no available pediatric dentists.

In Illinois, 752 residents died waiting for care due to the ACA's Medicaid expansion.

In a national survey after surgery, Medicaid recipients did no better than the uninsured, and thus billions of taxpayer dollars were wasted.[15] A study of Hepatitis C patients showed that Medicaid-covered patients often could not get the life-saving drugs they needed and they died.[16]

If you compare the process for medical care in the U.S. and single payer nations, we do better in some areas and worse in others.

Table 1-1: Comparison of U.S. Healthcare versus Single Payer Systems				
		Single Payer Systems		
Surrogate Metric of Quality	**U.S.**	**U.K.**	**Canada**	**Sweden**
Get timely care reminders	#3	#5	#9	#10
Reg. MD coordinates care	#3	#1	#4	#8
Reg. MD gives clear & complete instructions	#5*	#1	#5*	#11
Delays in notification	#9	#2	#11	#8
Reg. MD does *not* have sufficient information	#10	#7	#6	#11
Hospital follow-up care	#1	#2	#4	#8
Post-hospital communication with reg. MD	#3	#7*	#9	#7*
Overall timeliness of care	#5	#3	#11	#1
Wait ≥4 months for non-emergency surgery	#6	#4	#9	#5
U.S.=United States. U.K.=United Kingdom. Ranking (#) is from study of 11 industrialized nations; #1 is best and #11 is worst. Reg. MD=primary doctor. (*)=tied for position. GDP=gross domestic product. Source: "Mirror, Mirror on the Wall: How the Performance of the U.S. Health Care System Compares Internationally," published in June 2014.				

Some people use national longevity statistics as an indicator of success for a healthcare system. This is unwise. How long a large population lives is much more related to culture, diet, exercise, lifestyle, and genetics than to anything that doctors and nurses do for individual patients.

Fiscal Consequences

Though most commentators only discuss cost, and short-term cost at that, the measure we all should be using is *value*: benefits received for money expended. When calculating the value metric, the U.S. does poorly when compared to other countries. We are barely average in benefits received, and yet we spend double what most nations spend. Because we do not get double the benefits, the U.S. is not getting proper value for healthcare dollars expended.

When looking solely at cost, what was individually unaffordable before Obamacare is now even *more* unaffordable. (Editors say that more unaffordable is improper grammar. I left it that way because "more unaffordable" communicates quite clearly a reality we all face.) Until the real estate collapse of 2008–2009, medical bills constituted the #1 reason for filing personal bankruptcy in the U.S. Now, costs related to healthcare average 48 percent of a family's budget and are the biggest expense in the average family budget (See Table in the Introduction.)

The national fiscal picture is equally grim. In 1970, the U.S. was spending roughly the same amount per capita on healthcare as other developed nations. By 2010, we were spending more than double. Then, in 2010, we spent an additional $2 trillion for the ACA. How did that make healthcare "more affordable"?

We can also compare healthcare spending with a country's GDP. The higher the GDP, the richer a nation is. Figure 1-3 shows that most countries fall on a similar cost line, but there are two outliers, countries quite different from most others. First is Luxembourg, where people are very wealthy and spend only a moderate amount of their wealth on healthcare.

Then, there is the U.S., where individuals are moderately wealthy but spend much, much more on healthcare than anyone else.

Figure 1-3: U.S. Healthcare Spending Compared to Other Nations

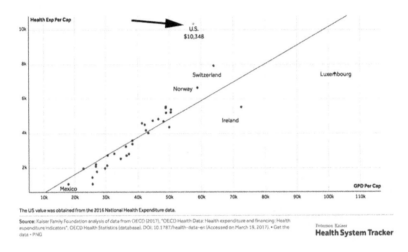

The US value was obtained from the 2016 National Health Expenditure data.

Source: Kaiser Family Foundation analysis of data from OECD (2017), "OECD Health Data: Health expenditure and financing: Health expenditure indicators", OECD Health Statistics (database). DOI: 10.1787/health-data-en (Accessed on March 19, 2017). • Get the data • PNG

Peterson Kaiser
Health System Tracker

The consequences of overspending on healthcare are worse for the states than for Washington for one obvious reason. The Treasury Department can print money—the states cannot. So, Texas may create budget allocations for 2018–2019, but Washington tells the Lone Star State how it is required by law to spend the first 30 percent of its budget.

The situation is even more grave (pun intended) for states like New Mexico, that expanded Medicaid under the ACA. Despite getting $3 billion shiny new federal dollars into the Land of Enchantment coffers, mandated costs of Medicaid were $3.4 billion. Thus, New Mexico Medicaid has a budget shortfall for 2017 of $417 million. To balance its budget, the state had to cut medical reimbursements to providers. Medicaid expansion gave more people insurance and left them with fewer service providers.

Senator Everett Dirksen is famous for an offhand remark, "a billion here, a billion there, and pretty soon you're talking real money!"[17] We are all aware that the U.S. is spending too much "real money" on healthcare. Where is it all going?

Are the insurance companies getting rich with their rent-seeking behaviors? There is some truth to that allegation. Others say the doctors and hospitals are the ones ripping us off. However, that is less true because the public thinks providers get paid what is written on the Bill for Services Rendered. In fact, providers are paid a fraction, often a very small fraction, of the price listed on the bill.

One way to answer the question of "Where does all the money go?" is to calculate dollar efficiency.[18] This measures the difference between money that goes into making something and the value a customer or end-user receives. For an auto manufacturer, dollar efficiency is the ratio of the cost to make the vehicle compared to the value that consumers perceive when buying the car.

In healthcare, dollar efficiency would be the amount of money spent compared to the quantity and quality of care patients receive. For simplicity, we can use "care received" as an indicator of quality and quantity. Thus, dollar efficiency in healthcare could be calculated as the amount of money we put into healthcare compared to how much care we get.

When you do that calculation, the minimum numbers for dollar efficiency are 60–69 percent meaning 31–40 percent of healthcare spending provides no care for patients.[19] Those estimates were made before Obamacare added nearly $2 trillion of additional bureaucratic expense. When you include cost of the ACA, dollar inefficiency in healthcare approches 50 percent. In simple terms, close to half of all our "healthcare" spending produces no care.

The answer to "Where does all that money go?" is to healthcare bureaucracy, administration, rules, regulations, and compliance. The money goes to the system, rather than the service. For a sense of perspective, we are wasting almost as much on healthcare bureaucracy as the entire country of Canada will produce in 2018: $1.79 trillion.

There are other, lesser-in-dollar-volume reasons for wasteful spending. Hundreds of millions of dollars are consumed by fraud and abuse as well as honest error. The regulations are impossibly complex, constantly changing, and often contradictory so that sometimes, it is simply impossible to comply with all the rules. The cost of defensive medicine has been estimated to be as high as $46 billion a year.[20] Finally, some over-spending is due to public expectations.

Before we conclude this first chapter, let's lighten the mood with a funny but real-world story. A woman brought a very limp duck into a veterinary surgeon. As she laid her pet on the table, the vet pulled out his stethoscope and listened to the bird's chest. After a moment or two, the vet shook his head sadly and said, "I'm sorry, your duck, Cuddles, has passed away." The distressed woman wailed, "Are you sure?"

"Yes, I am sure. The duck is dead," replied the vet. "How can you be so sure?" she protested. "I mean you haven't done any testing on him or anything. He might just be in a deep sleep or something." The vet rolled his eyes, turned around, and left the room.

He returned a few minutes later with a black Labrador Retriever. As the duck's owner looked on in amazement, the dog stood on his hind legs, put his front paws on the examination table, and sniffed the duck from top to bottom. He then looked up at the vet with sad eyes and shook his head from side to side. The vet patted the dog on the head and took it out of the room.

A few minutes later, he returned with a feline. The cat jumped on the table and also delicately sniffed the bird from head to tail. The cat sat back on its haunches, turned to the vet, shook its head, meowed softly, and strolled out of the room. The vet went to his computer, hit a few keys and produced a bill, which he handed to the woman. The duck's owner took the bill and read it.

"$250?!" she cried, "Just to tell me my duck is dead?" The vet shrugged, "I'm sorry. If you had just taken my word for it, the bill would have been $20, but with the Lab Report and the Cat Scan, it's now $250."

Conclusion

The U.S. healthcare system is clearly failing the American people. We can't get the care we need in time to save us from illness. We are spending more than we can afford and piling debt onto future generations.

As the late-night advertising heads shout from our TV sets, "But wait, "there's more!!" Isn't health care a right? And if it is, shouldn't everyone automatically get it, and for free? Let's explore this in the next chapter.

Chapter Notes

1. The "2013 Annual Report of the Boards of Trustees of the Federal Hospital Insurance and Federal Supplementary Medical Insurance Trust Funds,"

predicted that Medicare would be insolvent by 2030. A 2018 report revised that estimate to 2026. At that time, Medicare will be unable to provide care that seniors need. Note that even now, Medicare does not cover the most predictable and often necessary senior medical need: long-term nursing care.

2. The precise wording of Section 1801 of the 1965 Medicaid law is as follows: "Nothing in this title shall be construed to authorize any Federal officer or employee to exercise any supervision or control over the practice of medicine or the manner in which medical services are provided, or over the selection, tenure, or compensation of any officer or employee of any institution, agency, or person providing health services; or to exercise any supervision or control over the administration or operation of any such institution, agency, or person" See: Public Law 89–97, Hospital Insurance Program, 1965, page 291.

3. Mary Katherine Stout's 2006 paper, "Medicaid: Yesterday, Today, and Tomorrow: A Short History of Medicaid Policy and Its Impact on Texas" gives a vivid portrayal of the gradual, subtle, and incremental takeover of state Medicaid programs by the federal government, by giving the states their own tax revenue back. The states could have prevented this by simply "resisting federal blandishments," as suggested by Chief Justice Roberts in NFIB v. Sebelius in 2012. See the Healthcare Decoder in this book for more on the case.

4. Systems theory begins with the premise that a system, whether that *system* is a human body, a

corporation, or an entire industry like healthcare, succeeds or fails through the interaction of the parts of the system. No matter how good your heart is, you won't survive if your heart does not interact well with your kidneys, liver, and lungs. When there is a problem with one part of a system, fixing it without including the fix's effects on other organs often makes things worse, not better. Saving money in *Medicare* can make people sicker in *Medicaid*. Such a result is what systems thinkers call a fix-that-fails-or-backfires. This descriptor applies painfully well to what Congress has done repeatedly over the years to healthcare.

5. In *The Tragedy of American Compassion,* Marvin Olasky tells the compelling story of charitable activities in the U.S. It is sad to note that most of the lessons learned through that experience seem to have been lost in the current ascendancy of progressivism. At its height in the late 1950s, Cook County Hospital had more than 3,000 beds, served hundreds of thousands of indigent or impoverished residents of Chicago, and was one of the most sought-after training programs in the country.

6. The exact wording can be found in "Examination and treatment for emergency medical conditions and women in labor," Social Security Laws, Sec. 1867. [42 U.S.C. 1395dd]

7. In 2003, I analyzed the cost of uncompensated care for a major university hospital. Though the report was never published, it was made available at a meeting open to the public. The annual operating budget was

$960 million and the cost of uncompensated care was $235 million (24 percent).

8. See: "Privacy or Safety?" published by the Agency for Healthcare Research and Quality, July/August 2015.

9. The initial government estimate for the cost of Obamacare was $900 billion over ten years. It was later revised to $1.1 trillion, then $1.6 trillion, and eventually $2.6 trillion. The latest estimate is $1.76 trillion. Such wide variability of estimates indicates the limitations in Washington's ability to accurately predict true costs.

10. The designers of the ACA knew the law was incomprehensibly complex. So, they built into the law a requirement for states to hire "Navigators" to help patients find their way around through the maze of federal regulations, exceptions, exemptions, and legal language.

11. Merritt Hawkins is a national market research company that performed a survey in January and February 2017 titled, "2017 Survey of Physician Appointment Wait Times."

12. The Veterans Health Administration's 2015 report was titled, "Review of Alleged Mismanagement at the Health Eligibility Center."

13. Read what you need to know, which is more than you *want* to know, about death-by-queueing in *The Cancer in the American Healthcare System*.

14. The tragedy of Deamonte Driver was front-page news for weeks. Nick Horton originally reported the Illinois deaths online, but this too became a national print media sensation.

15. The study by Dr. Damien LaPar et al., "Primary Payer Status Affects Mortality for Major Surgical Operations," includes details of post-surgical results and death rates. The authors concluded, "Medicaid payer status was associated with the longest length of stay ... highest total costs ($P < 0.001$)," and an in-hospital mortality similar to those who were uninsured.

16. The Chief of Medicine at Inova Fairfax Hospital, Dr. Zobair Younossi, reported the findings on June 3, 2018 at a meeting of Digestive Disease Week.

17. According to Factchecker, no one could find proof that the late, great Senator from Illinois, ever uttered those words.

18. Years ago, I tried to write a song titled, "Where Has All the Money Gone?," using the 1950s Pete Seeger melody from "Where Have All the Flowers Gone?" I quickly learned how hard it is to be a lyricist.

19. In 2003, 11 years before all the ACA bureaucratic costs, Harvard researchers (Woolhandler et al., *New England Journal of Medicine*, 349:8) reported that bureaucracy consumed 31 percent of U.S. healthcare spending. In *The Cancer in the American Healthcare System* (2015), we reported that at least 40 percent was wasteful spending on bureaucracy. The ACA has certainly increased spending on bureaucracy.

20. "National Costs of the Medical Liability System" by Mello et al. in *Health Affairs* 2010 Sept.; 29(9):1569–1577. Most scientific articles are written to expose objective truth. Unfortunately, some are designed in advance to prove a point. Many cost analyses in

medicine, from both government and the academic community, fall into the latter category. I do not know if Mello's article is fact or spun data, but it was the best I could find. Consider it possible, even likely, while maintaining a small amount of skepticism as well.

Chapter 2:

Health Care *Cannot* Be a Right

What is healthcare? The answer depends on how it is spelled. As one word, *healthcare* refers to a complex industrial system that consumes close to 20 percent of U.S. gross domestic product (GDP). When *health care* is two words, it describes a legally protected, intimate, fiduciary relationship between a patient and physician. Health care is the work product of a professional that is purchased by a consumer, also known as a patient.

What is a right? The dictionary says a right is, "a moral or legal entitlement to have or obtain something or to act in a certain way." A right is an entitlement. You don't have to qualify for what you are entitled to, nor do you have to pay for it.

The First Amendment to the Constitution gives all Americans the right to free speech. No one needs to qualify. There is no test to pass or forms to fill out. There is no cost to speak your mind. Exercising a fundamental right is not a commercial activity.[1]

The founding document of the United States of America is the Declaration of Independence. It is much more than simply a declaration of war. It defined in clear and ringing terms that Americans' singular, highest, and most basic right is freedom.

Health care, as two words, **CANNOT** be a right, not in a country where the overarching right of all the people is freedom.

- ✓ Health care is a personal service that one person provides to another in exchange for money.
- ✓ If a person has a right to a provider's care, then the patient doesn't have to pay for that care.
- ✓ If a patient has a right to the personal service of a provider, then the provider is denied his or her freedom.
- ✓ If patients have a "right" to a provider's personal service—when, where, and whatever the patient wants—with no requirement for payment, that turns providers into slaves.

Figure 2-1: A Right to Health Care Turns Doctors into Slaves!

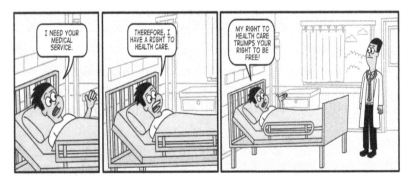

No Constitutional Basis for Federal Healthcare

Based on the Constitution, there are several reasons why healthcare should not be controlled by the federal government.

First, the Founding Fathers did not simply *forget* about health care: five of the signatories to the Declaration of Independence were physicians. Many more of the delegates to the Constitutional Convention were doctors.

Second, the Tenth Amendment clarifies the relationship between the federal government and the states. "The powers not delegated to the United States [meaning the federal government] by the Constitution, nor prohibited by it to the states, are reserved to the states respectively, or to the people." Thus, the federal government only has authority in the areas specified to it in the Constitution like "common defense," interstate commerce, and making our borders secure. Healthcare was never "delegated" to Washington. Therefore, healthcare is reserved "to the states respectively, or to the people."

The Commerce Clause in the Constitution was used as precedent to defend the ACA when challenged at the Supreme Court in 2012. [2] Yet nearly two hundred years earlier, the fourth Chief Justice of the U.S. Supreme Court, John Marshall, one of the staunchest upholders of the Constitution, wrote that "health laws of every description" are reserved exclusively to the states and not the federal government.[3]

It can't be much clearer than that who should be in charge of healthcare wherever you live: your state government, not Washington. That is true not just for Medicaid, but for all of the healthcare in your state.

There is a fourth, practical reason why federal control of healthcare is unconstitutional. A federal obligation to provide health care would require Washington to deny caregivers their freedom. How else would patients get care? What if no one wanted to go to medical or nursing schools? What if doctors refused to work for menial salaries? What if doctors wanted to practice medicine according to what they thought best for patients rather than how the government instructed them?

One American's "right" to receive care services from another American is anti-freedom, anti-American, and unconstitutional.

> When patients have a *right* to health care,
> doctors lose their right to be free.

Chapter Notes

1. If you reread the Bill of Rights, the first ten Amendments to the U.S. Constitution, the intent of our Founding Fathers becomes clear. All these Amendments are protection of individual freedom from the concentration of power that is called the federal government. The First Amendment says the government can't stop you from speaking your mind or praying however you wish, or not praying at all. The Third and Fourth Amendments say that you control your home and person, not the government. The Fifth through Eighth Amendments give you legal protections against a tyrannical government. And the Tenth Amendment very clearly limits the powers of the central authority.

2. The 2012 Supreme Court Case was *NFIB (National Federation of Independent Business) v. Sebelius,* who at that time was Secretary of Health and Human Services. The Court ruled that the Individual Mandate was unconstitutional, but it could be preserved if constituted as a tax. Two interesting notes: (1) In the NFIB case, the Obama administration argued that the individual mandate could not be severed from the rest of the law, as the whole structure of the law depended on it. In the 2017 Tax Reform bill,

Congress set the Obamacare individual "tax" at zero, meaning it generated no revenue and, thus, effectively ceased to exist. A lawsuit was filed in 2018 claiming that because the Obamacare regulations cannot be separated from the tax and the tax is null and void, then the whole law should be declared null and void. It may be years before this case reaches the Supreme Court; (2) In 2012, Chief Justice Roberts wrote that the states had a straightforward way to ignore federal healthcare mandates: they simply should "resist federal blandishments," meaning if they don't take federal money, they don't have to comply with federal rules.

3. John Marshall was Chief Justice of the U.S. Supreme Court from 1801 to 1835. He is considered one of the most influential legal thinkers in our nation's history. Writing about the use of the Commerce Clause in *Gibbons v. Ogden* (1824), Marshall said that the federal government has no business promulgating any health laws, period.

Chapter 3:

Healthcare Has Cancer

In the early part of the twentieth century, two events occurred that drove the cost of both health care and healthcare into the stratosphere. First, there were remarkable advances in medical technology. Doctors could treat conditions that were previously beyond their reach.

Cures became possible for infection, heart failure, and even cancer, but they were very expensive. Second, the rise of government-controlled healthcare and the development of the third-party payment structure eliminated the two free-market forces that keep prices down: buyers' incentive to economize and competition among sellers.

The great management guru, Russell Ackoff taught us there are four ways to fix a problem, whether it is a small matter or something as huge as our sick healthcare system.[1] You can absolve, solve, resolve, or dissolve a problem.

- Absolve means that you change nothing: you just forgive and forget.
- When solving a problem, you make things better than they currently are.
- Resolving a problem refers to making outcomes the best they can be *under the given circumstances.* Many

people confuse this with a cure. However, resolving leaves the root cause in place. The problem can recur.

- To <u>dissolve</u> a problem, you find the root cause and eliminate it. When the root cause is gone, all the symptoms—the bad results or outcomes—disappear.

When you resolve an issue, the problem can come back later or a new, related problem can appear. Dissolving is the best way to handle any difficulty. When the root cause ceases to exist, the symptoms cannot return. A brief explanation of diabetes highlights the distinctions between solve, resolve, and dissolve.

Diabetes is a problem with the regulation of glucose (sugar) in the body. Insulin is a molecule made in the pancreas that regulates how much glucose stays in the blood versus how much goes from the blood into the cells. When you have diabetes, you don't have enough insulin or the insulin you do have doesn't work right.

When you have diabetes, two bad things happen. The excess sugar in the blood makes you dehydrated and disturbs the balance of electrolytes in your blood. The lack of sugar inside the cells prevents organs like the liver, kidney, and heart from working properly. Acid builds up in the blood. If balance is not restored, you might die.

If you *solve* diabetes, you replace the lost water and electrolytes, give medicine to counteract the excess acid, and force the heart to work harder. If you *resolve* diabetes, you restore the proper amount of insulin in the blood. Resolving is the best we can do today. Medical science cannot (yet) dissolve or cure diabetes.

To *dissolve* or cure diabetes, first you must know the root cause or etiology. We do, sort of. There are specialized cells inside the pancreas that control the production of insulin. In diabetes, these cells do not work properly. That is the first half of the root cause, but the second half is unknown. Doctors do not know why these cells cease to function normally. When doctors learn what causes the pancreas cells to fail, they can help them return to good function. That will dissolve the root cause, and thus will CURE diabetes.

Curing diabetes is another medical miracle. I believe it will happen in my grandchildren's lifetime. I can absolutely guarantee it will be expensive. Most things of great value are.

A diagnosis for healthcare

The symptoms of healthcare system failure are obvious: national overspending, unaffordable care as well as unaffordable insurance, and inadequate access to care. What is the root cause, or what doctors call the etiologic diagnosis? We can find the answer by using a favorite mantra of forensic accountants: follow the money.

In 2017, the U.S. spent $3.5 trillion on healthcare. At least 40 percent, more than $1 trillion, was paid to support and expand federal bureaucracy, administration, rules, regulations, and compliance. The term that describes this phenomenon is *bureaucratic diversion.*[2] The result is too little money left after paying the bureaucracy to pay for care. See Figure 3-1 below.

Figure 3-1: Where Healthcare Dollars Go

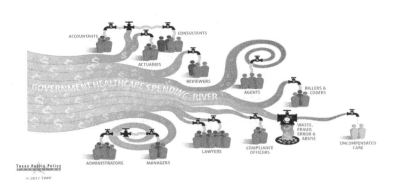

Between 1970 and 2010, the number of health care providers increased more than 100 percent, the grey area in Figure 3-2. Over the same 40 years, the number of healthcare bureaucrats grew by more than 3,000 percent. The data only goes as far as 2010: it does not include the further growth of bureaucracy induced by the Affordable Care Act.

Figure 3-2: Growth in Healthcare Bureaucrats and Doctors

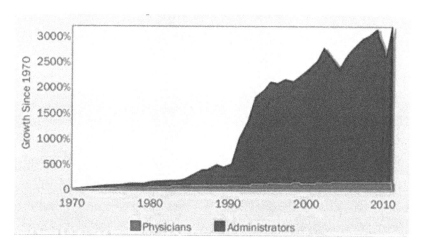

For a moment, ignore the question of whether healthcare really *needs* that number of bureaucrats and consider only the cost. In 2017, there were 953,000 licensed physicians in the U.S. The number of healthcare actuaries, accountants, administrators, agents, billers and coders, compliance officers, consultants, in-person assisters, lawyers, managers, navigators, regulators, reviewers, and rule writers in healthcare is not known but certainly is in the multi-millions. Furthermore, federal employees are more highly compensated, salary plus benefits, than those who do the same job in the private sector as in Figure 3-3.

Figure 3-3: Average Wages: Federal and Private Sector

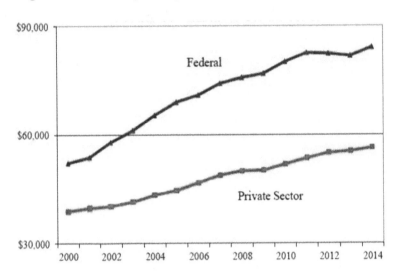

To paraphrase John Dunne's moving sermon from the mid 17th century that was immortalized by Ernest Hemingway's book, *For Whom the Bell Tolls,* "Never send to know to whom the money goes, it goes to ... *them.*"[3]

Taxpayers pay the costs for healthcare bureaucrats twice. First, taxpayers pay financially: bureaucrat salaries, benefits, pensions, overhead and other indirect costs. But, second and more important, taxpayers pay *medically* by reduced access to care. There is only a limited amount of healthcare dollars. Money paid to bureaucrats is money that cannot be spent on providers—bureaucratic diversion.

It is not simply fiscal cost of bureaucracy that hamstrings healthcare. In many ways the secondary "costs" of government are more harmful, especially long-term and particularly in the pharmaceutical world where the 800-pound gorilla is the FDA.

In 1962, Congress passed the Kefauver-Harris Amendments to the Food and Drug Act of 1938. While their intention was to secure a safe, reliable, effective supply of pharmaceutical agents, they turned the Federal Drug Agency into a Greek god, capricious, willful, often harming their "subjects" knowingly, and with essentially limitless power.[4] Watch how the federal bureaucracy put another nail in the coffin of new antibiotics.

The FDA has regulatory controls for every aspect of the pharmaceutical industry including planning, research, development, testing, manufacturing, even the packaging and especially the marketing. Their arduous and costly process has put a huge damper on the creation of new drugs, especially antibiotics. Between 1983 and 1987, the FDA approved 16 new antibiotics. In 2003 to 2007, despite the development of antibiotic resistant organisms, the FDA approved only five, and since then, zilch. Here's why.

Recall 2001 when two senators and several media offices were exposed to anthrax through the mail. Cipro (ciproflaxin) is an antibiotic primarily used for urinary tract infections, but it also kills anthrax. Bayer, the German pharmaceutical giant, was charging $2.00 a pill. The U.S. federal government wanted to stockpile 100 million pills, just in case. Congress did not want to pay $200 million for a "just in case," and so they browbeat the manufacturer to lower the price to $0.95 a pill.

At that time, Cipro was supposedly under patent protection. Bayer and every pharmaceutical manufacturer learned a bitter lesson: patent protection is meaningless when the federal government wants something. As a consequence, pharmaceutical manufacturers will be increasingly reluctant to develop new antibiotics and other drugs for that matter. If patents don't protect, how can they ever recover the massive costs that the FDA imposes.

To save $100 million, which is 0.005 percent of the cost of the ACA, we have prevented the next round of "wonder drugs."[5]

When the federal bureaucracy doesn't want to play by the rules, they just change them!

The Cipro story is just one of a host of examples of what happens when the government dictates the price of a product or service: you get less of it. Keep that in mind when someone (rightly) complains about the high price for drugs we need and then (wrongly) demands price controls. If the government drives down prices, you get shortages. If market competition drives down prices, you get more and better. Everyday examples would be Lasik surgery and mobile phones.

When I started as Chief of Pediatric Cardiology at the University of Chicago in 1990, I decided it would be a good idea for all of our senior team members to have up-to-date technology, i.e., mobile phones. Rapid, easy communication can be life-saving when dealing with critically ill newborn babies. (Selfishly, I wanted the hospital to be able to get ahold of me when I was out riding long miles training on my bike.)

Those were the days of the Hewlett Packard "brick" phones. They were the size and weight of a small brick and cost $3,500 each, retail. I gulped at the price and then went outside the University to shop around. I found a private vendor from whom I could get the phones for $1,700 each. While still concerned at the expense of buying six of them, I spoke with the University Procurement Officer and proudly gave her the good news that although I was spending $10,200, I was saving the department $10,800.

The officer condescendingly informed me that, "The university can't have its faculty going 'rogue' on them. There was a policy and procedure for procurement that had to be followed. If you want six of those phones, Dr. Waldman, I will get them."

And we did get them, at a cost of $21,000, doing it according to bureaucracy guidelines. Complying with the rules was more important than spending money wisely.

The diagnosis or root cause for healthcare system failure is clear: *Healthcare has cancer*. The cancer is an ever-expanding federal bureaucracy that controls us using the third-party payment structure. The cure would seem equally obvious. Apparently, that is not the case. Some believe the cure for excessive federal government control is … more government, more control, and, thus, more bureaucracy.

Chapter Notes

1. Russell L. Ackoff wrote several books and dozens of helpful articles. However, the best by far is his 1999, *Ackoff's Best: His Classic Writings on Management*. No matter what the reader does personally or professionally, there is much useful wisdom in this book. I urge everyone to read it (and no, I don't get a percentage of the proceeds.)

2. A whole chapter is needed to detail bureaucratic diversion in *"The Cancer in the American Healthcare System,"* another book worth your reading time.

3. John Dunne's phrase came from a sermon he wrote in 1624 when he was quite ill with what they called "spotted fever," which could have been any one of a host of viral or even bacterial diseases that cause high fever and skin eruptions. Fortunately, he recovered. While possibly at death's door, he wrote the following, "No man is an island, entire of itself; every man is a piece of the continent, a part of the main. If a clod be washed away by the sea, Europe is the less, as well as if a promontory were, as well as if a manor of thy friend's or of thine own were: any man's death diminishes me, because I am involved in mankind,

and therefore never send to know for whom the bells tolls; it tolls for thee."

4. Dr. Mary Ruwart's book, *Death by Regulation,* is a chilling tale of the history of the FDA. With solid evidence throughout, the author shows how one federal behemoth costs American lives, suppresses ingenuity and innovation, prevents release of treatments that could save us, and adds trillions (literally) to the price of drugs.

5. Prior to the development of antibiotics, infection was the leading cause of death, accounting for 30 percent of all U.S. deaths in 1900. The creation of ever more powerful, broad spectrum antibiotics dropped the death rate from infection by 95 percent between 1900 and 1980. That is why they were called "wonder drugs." Sadly, we have become blasé about these potent medicines. While we were sleeping, bacteria have developed resistant strains to tuberculosis, staphylococcus, and other dangerous germs. With the FDA suppressing new drug development, epidemiologists and clinical physicians have grave concerns.

Chapter 4:

Single Payer Is Poison, Not Panacea

S ome people believe the cure for the sick U.S. healthcare is single payer. They have obviously not read, *Single Payer Won't Save Us.*[1] If they had seen that compilation of evidence about single payer systems both in the U.S. and abroad, they would know it is poison for patients, not panacea.[2]

Figure 4-1: Some People Want Single Payer Healthcare in the U.S.

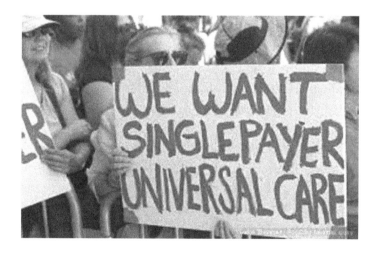

Advocates believe the following three claims (falsehoods) regarding single payer healthcare systems. Rather than deciding on faith or being persuaded by others' passion, consider the facts.

Single Payer Falsehoods

1. Single payer has been proven to work.

Have you ever heard of doctors going on strike here in the U.S.? In 2016, British doctors who work for the vaunted National Health Service (NHS) went out on strike, twice.[3] Further, the British High Court has declared that in life-or-death medical decisions, the hospital can override the family's wishes. That is not what Americans call an effective, a "working," much less a compassionate system, and, there's worse, much worse, news about single payer.

The single payer NHS, touted by President Obama and ACA architects, is actually medically dangerous. Despite numerous reports of inappropriate care and avoidable deaths, "when the state is a monopoly provider of health care, there is a political interest in suppressing bad news" (such as unnecessary deaths) despite the public's right, indeed, *need* to know. [4]

The single payer system in England tried to use death-by-queueing on my Mum, but we foiled them!

I had two mothers. My natural mother, Mom, was American. My adoptive mother, Mum, was British. She lived just outside Liverpool and worked as a midwife. Of course, she was enrolled in the NHS. When she fell and broke her hip, we assumed the healthcare system would fix it. She was told that she could have hip replacement surgery but had to wait in line until her turn— 27 months in the future!

If a 78-year-old, overweight woman were forced to remain immobilized in bed for more than two years, she would likely develop pneumonia, become obese, watch her muscles atrophy, probably have a blood clot in the lungs (pulmonary embolus), and die long before her surgery. Death-by-queueing.

I discussed this with my British brother, Stewart. I suggested a letter to the NHS requesting prompt surgery on medical grounds for the patient's best interest. Stewart said appealing to altruism wouldn't work, but a financial argument might be heard. Stewart was Editor of the *Financial Times* so, he naturally leaned toward the fiscal side.

I composed a letter containing two cost analyses for the NHS: surgery now or surgery in 27 months. (My MBA came in handy.) The former essentially was the expense of the procedure and post-operative rehabilitation. The latter included all the nursing costs, additional medical expenses, and assistive devices for a bed-ridden patient until surgery, plus the operation followed by rehabilitation. Mum had her surgery two months later, went back to work, and lived for another seventeen years.

In Canada's single payer system, patients experience death-by-queueing.[5] A Canadian surgeon Dr. Ciaran McNamee, sued the Provincial government of Alberta, claiming he had numerous medical records that proved Canadians died waiting in line for care. The fatal delays occurred because their central government restricts allocations for medical equipment and services. There were too few burn units to care for burn victims, and too few surgical suites to operate in time to save patients.

Medicaid, though it functions through middlemen insurance companies, also has elements of single payer systems, such as government mandates that determine what care people get and how much providers will be paid. The following describes what Medicaid did to patients.

- **For Want of a Dentist:** In Chapter 1, there was the story of Deamonte Driver who was eligible for government coverage but never got care. While Medicaid is not a typical single payer structure, it is government-controlled healthcare that does not produce adequate access to timely care. As a result, a 12-year-old boy died needlessly and avoidably from complications of an untreated tooth cavity.

- **Death by Waiting:** Illinois expanded its Medicaid program under the ACA. As happened in New Mexico, as noted in Chapter 1, expansion increased the number of insured individuals and at the same time increased the wait time for care. Nicholas Horton[6] showed that as a result, 752 Illinoisans died while *in queue.*

- **More Medicaid ≠ Better Health:** A study of Medicaid expansion in Oregon[7] showed that Medicaid patients felt less anxious because they had insurance coverage. However, their health outcomes were no better than those who had no insurance at all. Taxpayers paid billions to relieve the worries of Medicaid enrollees but did not improve their physical health.

Studies of healthcare system quality should include individual health outcomes such as cardiac function after heart surgery or mobility after a hip replacement, but most do not. Instead, they use surrogate measures of quality, such as complication rates and communication adequacy. As shown in Chapter I, Table 1-1, the Commonwealth Fund[8] found that single payer systems were sometimes better than the U.S., and in other respects, they were not.

2. Single payer systems spend much less than the U.S.

Single payer systems are, in fact, cheaper *for their countries* than the U.S., as shown in Table 4-1. Whether you consider national spending per capita or as a percentage of GDP, the U.S. expends much more on healthcare than other nations.

Table 4-1 National Healthcare Spending		
Country	**% GDP**	*per capita*
Canada (SP)	10.9	$4,608
Finland (SP)	9.4	$3,984
Italy (SP)	9.1	$3,272
Japan (SP)	10.3	$4,150
Sweden (SP)	8.8	$5,228
Spain (SP)	8.9	$3,153
UK (SP)	9.1	$4,003
U.S.	17.2	$9,451
SP=Single Payer. GDP=gross domestic product. UK=United Kingdom		

However, when it comes to spending by *individuals or families*, national comparisons become confusing. Both how people spend money and how spending is accounted vary greatly from country to country. In the U.S., payments are made to insurance carriers by individuals or families, or for them by employers or by the government through Medicaid. In 2018, the average

American family spent $28,166 on healthcare. That represented 44 percent of their income before taxes.

The tax burden in single payer countries is higher than the U.S. What is not known is how much of the taxes paid by a Briton, a Swede, or a Canadian was consumed by their single payer healthcare system.

Attempts to study healthcare financing in both single payer nations and the U.S. discover an opaque—the opposite of transparent—system, where it is virtually impossible to follow the money trail. This is not by accident. Governments do not want people to know precisely where their money is going.

How do single payer systems spend less money than the U.S.? By rationing, two different ways. Government allocates the amount to be spent on operating rooms or burn units. Such spending is not based on patient needs but on budgetary constraints. Therefore, many burn victims cannot get specialized burn care and some people needing surgery die waiting for an available operating suite.

Figure 4-2: There Is Good News ... and Bad

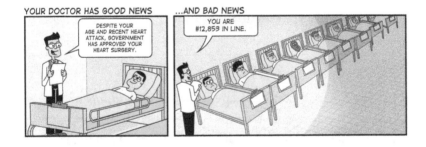

Single payers also ration care by what they authorize for payment versus what they classify as "Not Cost Effective" and then refuse to authorize. The latter is unavailable even though treatment might save the patient's life.

For example, Great Britain sets age limits on treatments and procedures, such as kidney dialysis and heart surgery. If you are too old, the treatment is not authorized. Unless you can pay $125,000 for your coronary bypass or $10,000 per month for dialysis, you die. That is how and why #3 below is *not* true.

3. Everyone gets the care they need with single payer.

Supporters of single payer claim that everyone gets the care they need. This is patently false because of strict medical rationing.

In Great Britain, there is an agency that has the most misleading abbreviation I have ever read. N.I.C.E., the National Institute for Clinical Excellence, is anything but nice. This agency is tasked with deciding what treatments will be authorized and which will not. Those not authorized for payment effectively become unavailable because only the very expensive ones are rejected by N.I.C.E., and people cannot afford them.

Figure 4-3: Single Payers Are Cheaper Because They Ration Medical Care

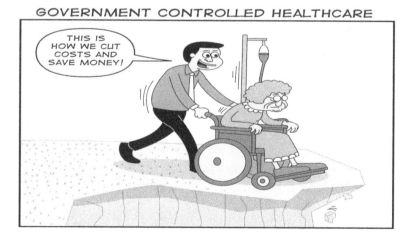

A good example is kidney dialysis, which costs more than $10,000 per month in the U.S. In Great Britain's single payer, kidney dialysis over age 55 years was deemed "Not Cost Effective," and authorization was denied to those over 55. This simple rationing approach did save money at the *cost* of people's lives. Britons died who could have been saved.

Government control is the reason healthcare is failing patients everywhere. And single payer devotees advocate a system where the government has total control!

The current overregulated structure is wasting our money and denying us the care we need. Yet, single payer advocates believe the answer is more regulations.

Government healthcare is poison. Increasing the dose of poison is not good for We the Patients.

A homegrown single payer

We can observe single payer's bad medical outcomes without ever leaving the U.S. Just look at one of our homegrown single payer systems: the Veterans Health Administration system, or VA.

Start with the worst: death-by-queueing. As noted in Chapter 1, an internal VA audit of patient outcomes concluded that, "307,000 veterans may have died waiting for approval for medical care."

Then there are VA nursing homes. A 2018 expose of VA nursing home care shows not only that single payer VA facilities provide substandard care, but the single payer, i.e., the federal government, covers it up just like the single payer NHS in Great Britain.

The Centers for Medicare and Medicaid Services (CMS) oversees the care provided to elders in nursing homes, both private and VA. The facilities are required to submit reports with all types of quality measures, such as pain levels, amounts of drugs prescribed, bed sores, hospitalizations and re-admissions, infection rates, and deaths. Data from the private facilities is available on a public website. The VA does not share its data with anyone, not even Congress.[10]

In June 2018, reporters from *USA Today* and the *Boston Globe* obtained the embargoed data on quality results in VA nursing homes. Their investigative report showed that for ten of eleven measures of quality, residents in VA nursing homes through the country consistently did worse that residents in private facilities.[11]

The Acting Secretary of the VA, Peter O'Rourke, released a statement calling the report by *USA Today* and the *Boston Globe* "fake news." Then, he refused to release the data that he said would prove his point.

Single payers fail to provide adequate care and then hide their inadequacies.

A cure that will work

Federal control of healthcare is the root cause of system sickness. The cure for Patient Healthcare is not more federal control, i.e., single payer, but the precise opposite: *Get Washington out of healthcare.*

What does "get Washington out of healthcare" look like?

Chapter Notes

1. When released, *Single Payer Won't Save Us* was #4 on the Amazon bestseller list.
2. Panacea comes from Greek mythology: Panacea was the goddess of universal remedy, a cure-all for

everything from a cut finger to cancer. Panacea was the daughter of Epione, the goddess of soothing pain, and Asclepius, son of Apollo and god of healing arts. Another daughter they had was Hygieia. From her name we get the word, hygiene.

3. In April 2016, *U.S. News & World Report* reported, "Thousands of doctors have posted picket lines outside hospitals around England in the first all-out strike in the history of the National Health Service."

4. The following are some of the reports that document scandalous medical outcomes in the NHS: Bristol Royal Infirmary Inquiry, 1994; "Top doctor's chilling claim: The NHS kills off 130,000 elderly patients every year" in *The Daily Mail*, 2012; Morecambe Bay Hospital Report, 2015; "Single-Payer in Crisis: Britain's NHS Cancels 50,000 Surgeries Amid Long Waits For Care, 'Third World' Conditions" in Townhall, 2018; Gosport Independent Panel, June 2018; "Great Britain Offers Cautionary Tale on Single Payer" in *RealClear Health*, 2018; and "Reform the NHS Before It Kills Again" in *The Wall Street Journal*, 2018.

5. See chapters 8 and 9 in *The Cancer in the American Healthcare System*.

6. In 2016, Horton published "Hundreds on Medicaid Waiting List in Illinois Die While Waiting for Care."

7. The research done on Oregon's "natural social experiment" was published in 2013 in the *New England Journal of Medicine* titled, "The Oregon Experiment—Effects of Medicaid on Clinical Outcomes."

8. The Commonwealth Fund report, "Mirror, Mirror on the Wall: How the Performance of the U.S.

Health Care System Compares Internationally" was published in June 2014.

9. See Woolhandler, et al., "Costs of Health Care Administration in the United States and Canada." *The New England Journal of Medicine,* 349.8 (August 21, 2003): 768–775.

10. Following the *USA Today/Boston Globe* exposé, two Senators, Bill Cassidy (R-LA) and Doug Jones (D-AL) had to introduce legislation that would force the VA to release all of its nursing home quality information.

11. The report by Slack and Estes not only summarized the findings, but provided the public with the actual VA data, clearly disproving Acting VA Secretary O'Rourke's assertion that their report was false ("fake news").

Chapter 5:

The Cure – *StatesCare*

With the root cause of healthcare failure clearly in mind[1], cancer, the fix or cure is straightforward: remove the cancer. Since the root cause is an overgrown, overbearing, massively overspending federal bureaucracy, the cure is to cut down the bureaucracy to a manageable size. But how can this be done? Some say it is impossible. If you agree that healthcare cannot be fixed, you guarantee that it never will be fixed. You have created a self-fulfilling prophecy.

If we wait for Washington to fix healthcare, we will be waiting forever. It was Washington that created and continuously expanded its healthcare bureaucracy. Federal politicians are either unwilling or unable to accept the truth. They, their rules, their regulations and mandates are the problem. Therefore, they, their rules, their regulations, and mandates can never be the solution.

Consider the federal mandates as though they are ballast on the gondola of a hot air balloon before Obamacare, with a limited number of people having free insurance and a number of mandates. The hot air balloon could get off the ground, but barely (See the left-side balloon in Figure 5-2).

Figure 5-1: Mandates Piled on Top of Mandates on Top of Mandates

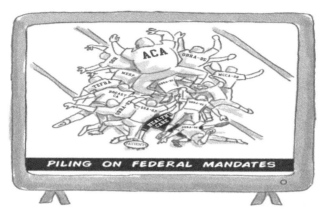

The Affordable Care Act gave no-charge Medicaid insurance to an additional 17 million Americans, thus adding more people to the gondola under the balloon. The ACA also added a host of new rules and regulations—mandates—to healthcare. As indicated by the middle balloon, it can't even get off the ground.

Figure 5-2: Can the Healthcare Balloon Soar?

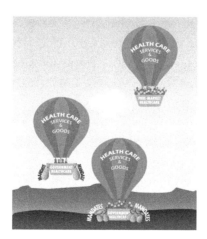

But take away the mandates and release the free market, and as shown by the right-side balloon (Figure 5-2), healthcare can soar, meaning it can actually provide needed care to all Americans. All we have to do is free healthcare from federal control-by-mandate.

Chief Justice Roberts wrote that federal Medicaid mandates, "undermine the status of the States as independent sovereigns in our federal system." And in the landmark NFIB case that upheld Obamacare, Justice Roberts noted, "... we look to the States to defend their prerogatives by adopting 'the simple expedient of not yielding' to federal blandishments (money) when they do not want to embrace the federal policies as their own."[2] If a state doesn't like federal Medicaid mandates, states shouldn't take federal Medicaid money.

Washington is reluctant to give up control of one sixth of our economy to the states. Malignant expansion of the federal bureaucracy creates loyal federal bureaucrats who support Washington, vote for the people who gave them jobs, and will resist anything that makes their well-paying jobs go away.[3]

Some might claim reluctance to give up federal power is limited to progressives or to Democrats. Not true. While Republicans claim they want to reduce the size of government, they never do it. Ronald Reagan, a paragon of conservatives, expanded the size of the federal government.[4] It was Republicans who passed HIPAA. It was Republicans who did not repeal Obamacare when they had the chance in 2017.

Both major political parties have the same strategic approach to all problems in healthcare: expand the power of the federal government by increasing the size, scope, reach, and expense of its handmaiden bureaucracy.

Strategic plan

Many people believe strategic planning is only for military operations. In fact, every time you want to do anything, from manufacturing a car to hiring a new employee to buying a candy bar, you need a strategic plan to accomplish your goal.

Curing the cancer in healthcare is what we want to accomplish. So, we need a strategic plan. The first step is to decide on the objective, the result you want. As Stephen Covey advised everyone, "Start with the end in mind." The "end," the desired outcome, should be what you truly want, not what you think is practicable or realistic.

America was built on the idea that *Americans can do anything.* Freedom combined with capitalism releases our potential. Anything is possible, including a healthcare system that works, meaning a system that provides **timely, quality health care chosen by the patient at a cost that both individuals and the nation can afford**.

THAT is the "end" we want. THAT is the goal of our strategic plan.

Both managers and doctors have a similar piece of wisdom on the timing of implementing a strategic plan. Physicians know the sicker a patient is, the faster you must heal him. Managers know that the more radical the change that is needed, the faster you should make it happen. If you do things very slowly, incrementally, while avoiding any shocks to the system, the forces of status quo, who oppose any change, will become more organized and stop the cure. In the ER, if you do things very slowly, incrementally, while avoiding any shocks, the auto accident victim will die.

In other words, a massive change like getting the federal government out of healthcare, should be accomplished over years, not generations. And never confuse an intermediate step along the way as the final outcome.

A good strategy enlists the people involved rather than being imposed on them from above. That is particularly true of Americans. We expect to rely on ourselves. We prize our freedom over goodies the government promises to deliver, but never does. "A government big enough to give you everything you want, is a government big enough to take away everything that you have."[5] One reason people resist Obamacare is the fact that President Obama imposed his namesake law on citizens against our will. Even if it were "for our own good" (it isn't), we still would resist because it denies our freedom. And, of course, lawmakers did not impose Obamacare on themselves; lawmakers made themselves exempt from it for good reason. They knew the whole thing was rotten.

So, while a strategy for radical change must move quickly, Americans must be involved in the development, engaged in the process, educated about what it means to them personally, and enthusiastic for what is going to happen.

A problem is only truly fixed when the root cause is gone. For healthcare, curing the cancer means getting Washington out of healthcare. That means healthcare decisions should be made by the people in their states, not by Washington politicos and bureaucrats. That is what we call *StatesCare*.[6]

StatesCare transfers the organization, financing, administration, and regulation (what little is necessary) of healthcare to state legislatures. Representing their people, state legislators decide the healthcare structure best suited to their people's needs and state resources.

If Californians want a single payer system, they should be allowed to "chart their own course," as urged by state Senator Richard Lara.[7] Washington should not simply say No. If Texas wants to create a market-based system, that should be the Lone Star State's choice. Do not get sucked into the argument that

Washington is giving the states *their* (Washington's) money. Washington only has money that the people give it. The states want to spend their tax dollars that they allocate to healthcare as they see fit, not as a federal bureaucrat decides.

There may be incremental, intermediate steps along the way to getting Washington totally out of healthcare, but the end goal should always be in mind. We probably have to use ju-jitsu rather than a nuclear weapon.

It is unlikely that Washington will easily relinquish authority over healthcare to the states until there is a massive groundswell felt at the ballot box and/or a Convention of States.[8] Until those events occur, there is something the states can do—by starting with the "800-pound gorilla" in healthcare: Medicaid.

Waivers

Most federal legislative acts, no matter the specific content, contain a process by which a state can request a variance from what the law says. This process is called a waiver and is intended to allow the state to demonstrate that an alternative approach, different from what the law mandates, will achieve better results. Waivers are generally named for their section numbers within the law.

For example, the original Medicaid law of 1965 has Section 1115 that allows a state to waive federal regulations the state specifies in the waiver request. All waivers must be approved by the relevant federal agency. For healthcare, that is the Centers for Medicare & Medicaid Services (CMS).

Medicaid programs are failing in 50 states and the District of Columbia—that's Washington D.C. where all those legislators are supposed to be "fixing" healthcare. These programs are devouring state resources,[9] restricting access,[10] and sometimes showing worse medical outcomes than being uninsured.[11]

Part of the reason for these failures is distortion of the original goals of Medicaid. Conceived as a program for those who are "unable," i.e., aged, blind, and disabled, and not merely the poor. Intended for those who would literally die without government support for their medical care, Medicaid now covers perfectly healthy, able-bodied person up through 25 years of age.

Medicaid law established programs that were supposed to be state-administered. Piece by piece, new rules altered more rules, and administrative functions have been co-opted by Washington, from eligibility standards and verification processes to benefit packages and even pricing. A partial list of the bills that contained Medicaid mandates includes Social Security Amendments of 1967; Omnibus Budget Reconciliation Acts (OBRA) of 1981, 1985, 1987, 1989, 1990, and 1993; Balanced Budget Act of 1997; Deficit Reduction Act of 2005; and, of course, the ACA.[12]

Chapter 537

In 2011, Texas started on the road to fixing Texas Medicaid by passing Chapter 537 into state law. This chapter was a request for a total waiver of Medicaid mandates plus a block grant for support. The waiver request was never submitted to CMS. It remains as state law that has not been activated.

Keep in mind the year, 2011. The ACA had been passed in 2010 and was still being modified almost on a daily basis. No one knew what the final law would be and no one knew what its effects would be. Further, the ACA was not implemented until January of 2014. Thus, in 2011, there was no evidence-of-effect for Obamacare.

Therefore in 2012, the Texas Legislative Oversight Committee, taking into account the political climate of the time, chose not to move the waiver request to CMS. Chapter 537 remains in Texas government code to this day, but it has not been enacted.

The time to apply Chapter 537 is now, 2018. President Trump's very first executive order, signed two hours after he took office, encouraged federal agencies to do whatever they could to give the states a free hand in healthcare.[13] The new Director of CMS, Seema Verma, has repeatedly said that she will not tell the states what to do or what waivers to seek: she wants the states to come to CMS with their ideas.

As a block grant and waiver of all mandates, Chapter 537 will return administrative control of Texas Medicaid to where it belongs: Texas. The same would be true for any other state that received approval for a similar waiver request.

Figure 5-3: A Waiver Can Restore Control to Texas, Temporarily

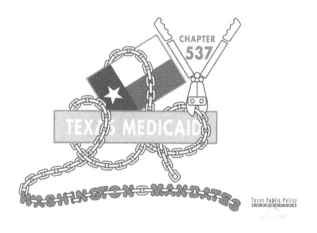

While states might start with Medicaid waivers, the goal is the same, *StatesCare*, Let the States Decide. A state can choose to go it alone. States can form alliances or regional coalitions and choose a system for the group. If a state or a coalition wants Obamacare, it is free to select that approach.

Keep in mind that, compared to Washington bureaucrats, state legislators are more knowledgeable about local needs and local resources, and are much more in contact with their constituents. If voters do not like the system that their legislators propose, the legislators will quickly find out at the ballot box. In fact, voters are much more likely to be involved in the creation of a state system when their state representative, who lives next door and uses the same barber shop, is the one who will help create it.

Some California legislators and advocacy groups there want a single payer structure for their 39 million residents. While the evidence suggests *to me* that single payer is a flawed concept,[14] my opinion should carry the same weight in California as what Washington lawmakers think—none! California should decide what is best for California. That is what *StatesCare* is all about— let each state decide for itself.

Texas believes that a market-based healthcare system is most likely to achieve Lone Star State goals for its people. Can a free market approach work in healthcare? Some say yes. Others say no. What are the facts? Read on.

Always keep in mind, if you live in Rhode Island and don't like either California's or Texas's plans, you do not have to follow their lead. This is *StatesCare*—you and your state decide what system you want. No one tells you what system you must have.

Legal basis for *StatesCare*

The Tenth Amendment to the U.S. Constitution reads, "The powers not delegated to the United States by the Constitution, nor prohibited by it to the States, are reserved to the States respectively, or to the people." Healthcare was not a power delegated to the federal government and, thus, was reserved to the states and the people.

The Founding Fathers of our country did not simply "forget" about healthcare. Five signatories on the Declaration of Independence as well as numerous delegates to the Constitutional Convention were physicians.

State or popular control of healthcare was reiterated by the great jurist, Chief Justice John Marshall in 1824 (*Gibbon v. Ogden*): "health laws of every description" are reserved to the states.

Section 1801 of the 1965 Medicaid law is titled, "Prohibition against any federal interference." The authors clearly intended for all Medicaid programs to be administered locally, i.e., by the states. However, over five decades, the federal government has taken over every aspect of 51 Medicaid programs using a one-size-fits-all approach.[15]

Figure 5-4: Washington: Get Out of Texas Medicaid

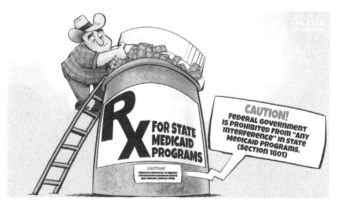

In 2012, even as he upheld the Obamacare law from legal challenge, Chief Justice Roberts reminded us that states are "sovereign entities" that can choose to ignore federal healthcare mandates by simply "resisting federal blandishments."

Even though the waiver process may be the most politically viable option, many Americans recoil from the necessity. They believe the individual, not the government, should be able to decide his or her own health care and one should not have to ask permission from Washington to exercise a freedom that should have been theirs in the first place.

If *StatesCare* were available to the Lone Star State, what would Texas do with this freedom?

Chapter Notes

1. For the complete explanation from symptoms to diagnosis of root cause, read *The Cancer in the American Healthcare System*.
2. The quote can be found on page 49 of "National Federation of Independent Business v. Sebelius, Secretary of Health and Human Services," No. 11–393, June 28, 2012.
3. Federal bureaucrats are paid 78 percent more than private sector workers. In 2014, federal compensation averaged $119,934, while average income in the private sector was $67,246.
4. There is debate on this issue depending on an author's political bias. Reagan's detractors say that spending increased, while his supporters point to his taking authority from the bureaucratic "state" and returning them to the legislative branch.
5. Like many individuals, I thought Thomas Jefferson said this. Apparently, I was wrong. The first appearance of this quote was found in Paul Harvey's 1952 book, *Remember These Things*, 126 years after the death of Jefferson.

6. For a while, we have been suggesting the concept of *StatesCare* in different ways in various publications, such as:
   - *The Hill*, Nov. 12, 2016. "The Great Disruptor Can Fix Healthcare."
   - *FoxNews.com*, Jan. 4, 2017. "A Doctor's Straight Talk: America, Your Health Care Is Not a Federal Responsibility."
   - *Washington Examiner*, March 23, 2017. "Instead of the House Healthcare Bill, Replace Federal Healthcare Laws by Letting the States Decide What to Do."
   - *The Daily Caller*, May 4, 2017. "Let States Have Their Own Healthcare Systems."
   - *The Hill*, Nov. 30, 2017. "ObamaCare Contributed to the Murder of Health Care, But It's Not the Only Culprit."

7. Another time the *StatesCare* idea appeared in print was in, "California and Texas Agree on Health Care," in *Real Clear Health*, June 2017.

8. Article 5 of the U.S. Constitution shows how the people can force a recalcitrant Congress to do what the people want. It reads as follows. "The Congress ... shall propose Amendments to this Constitution, or, on the *Application of the Legislatures of two thirds of the several States*, [italics added for emphasis] shall call a Convention for proposing Amendments, which ... shall be valid to all Intents and Purpose." With current Congressional approval ratings hovering in the teens, enthusiasm for a Convention of States is increasing. In fact, as of January 2018, 27 states have passed resolutions

calling for redress of government overreach using Article 5. When the number of states reaches 34, a Convention will be called, according to our Constitution.

9. Read how Medicaid spending is consuming Texas resources that are needed for education, infrastructure, or border security in, "The Saga of 1115—A Waiver Can Fix Texas Medicaid, But Only Temporarily," published March 2017.

10. A 2017 survey by Merritt Hawkins showed that expansion of the people on Medicaid by the ACA increased the wait time to see a family physician by more than four months!

11. A national study of nearly a million people after surgery demonstrated worse outcomes and higher costs in Medicaid-covered patients.

12. See "ObamaCare contributed to the murder of health care, but it's not the only culprit," *The Hill*, November 2017.

13. The exact wording of President Trump's Executive Order #1 is as follows: "…executive departments and agencies with authorities and responsibilities under the Act [the Affordable Care Act] … shall exercise all authority and discretion available to them to waive, defer, grant exemptions from, or delay the implementation of any provision or requirement of the Act that would impose a fiscal burden on any State …"

14. I wrote an eBook on the subject titled, "*Single Payer Won't Save Us.*" I suspect that people who advocate single payer for the U.S. have never read this book. They really need to.

15. Mary Katherine Stout's 2006 paper, "Medicaid: Yesterday, Today, and Tomorrow—A Short History of Medicaid Policy and Its Impact on Texas," details the piece by piece takeover by Washington of all U.S. "state" Medicaid programs.

Chapter 6:

The Texas Model

O ptions for curing healthcare in Texas do *not* begin by asking what is practical or likely to get Congressional approval. Political expedience is not a proper starting point to achieve a cure, whether the patient is a sick person or a failing healthcare system.

Stephen Covey always said, "Start with the end in mind." The goal of any cure for healthcare is a system where Americans are free to choose their own caregivers and their own care; free to decide whether to spend their money or not, and on what; and free from the interposition of a third party, whether government or insurance carrier, between patient and doctor.

Washington has been likened to a swamp that controls both us as individuals and our healthcare system. If we dissolve the root cause, if we take away control of healthcare from the federal government, then who should be in charge? Clearly, the people and the states.[1] Healthcare structured by the states but with patients in charge of themselves is what we call *StatesCare*.[2]

What should states do with their newfound, or more accurately, finally-restored Tenth Amendment independence? They should do whatever they think best for their own people, knowing the local needs and available resources much better than a central authority.

Research shows that third-party payment structure is largely to blame for healthcare system failure. The solution is, therefore, to remove the third-party payment structure. What might healthcare look like with the feds out and market forces replacing third-party payment?

It could be as simple as ... *TexasCares*, a market-based healthcare system with a safety net for the medically vulnerable. Such a system could achieve the **best, timeliest care at the lowest price** for 29 million Texans. Just imagine what that could do for every state and millions more people across the country!

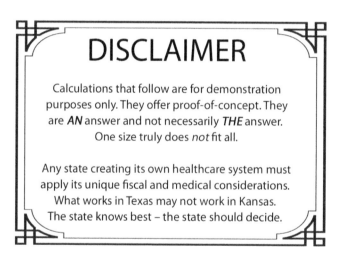

DISCLAIMER

Calculations that follow are for demonstration purposes only. They offer proof-of-concept. They are **AN** answer and not necessarily **THE** answer. One size truly does *not* fit all.

Any state creating its own healthcare system must apply its unique fiscal and medical considerations. What works in Texas may not work in Kansas. The state knows best – the state should decide.

Principles for Texas Healthcare

The United States of America replaced a failing, centrally controlled *political system* with one based on personal liberty. To replace a failing, centrally controlled *healthcare system,* Texas would do well to follow our Founding Fathers and start by enunciating foundational principles. The following are foundational tenets for a new, Lone Star healthcare system named *TexasCares.*

✓ FREEDOM: Healthcare must not impinge on the liberty of Texans.

✓ PERSONAL RESPONSIBILITY: With freedom comes personal responsibility, always.

✓ HEALTH: Good health requires the patient to be responsible, not the government nor the doctor.

✓ PROSPERITY: Good health is a prerequisite to personal prosperity: material comfort, security, and self-actualization.

✓ DOLLAR EFFICIENCY: *TexasCares* must be dollar efficient, devoting the most funds to care and the least to non-care activities such as administration and bureaucracy.

✓ PRIORITIZATION: Texas should be free to prioritize all state spending as Texas sees fit.

Texas Medicaid was chosen as the place to demonstrate the effectiveness of the Texas model. Medicaid is a paradigm of government-controlled, third-party payment healthcare. It also includes some of the sickest Americans. If conversion to a free market can work in Medicaid, it can work anywhere.

In 2017, the CEO of a medium-sized Texas company called the main desk at the Texas Public Policy Foundation demanding "to speak with someone who knew what in blazes is going on with healthcare and who could do something about it!" The intern immediately called my office and hesitantly asked if I would speak with the caller. Of course, I said, "Yes."

When we were connected, he asked who I was and then without waiting for an answer, he began regaling me with complaints told to him by several of his employees. One employee got a surprise bill after an ER visit at a facility where his costs were supposedly covered by his health plan. Another employee had a child whose doctor wanted a second opinion, but the insurance company kept giving excuses why this could not be done. A third employee needed a medication prescribed by her doctor but the Pharmacy Benefits Manager repeatedly denied prescriptions written by the doctor.

The CEO continued, "Why am I paying all this money to insurance companies if my people can't get the care they need? Am I just throwing hundreds of thousands of dollars in the toilet?!"

After taking two deep, cleansing breaths, (I shared his outrage but had to sound calm), I began to explain. "Healthcare has a third-party payment and not the free market we are used to. The third-party insurance company that pays for goods and services has a strong incentive *not* to provide service. That is why they delay, defer, or deny care," I continued.

When I began to show how this explained his employees' experiences, he again interrupted me exclaiming, "That's the dumbest thing I ever heard! Who invented such a stupid system," he asked? "Congress," I replied. And then, without knowing anything about systems theory, good medical practice, and lacking my years of studying and analyzing our healthcare system, the CEO came up with the perfect answer.

"Hell, son, that's easy. Texas should just tell Washington to ***crude-expletives-and-anatomically-impossible-requests-deleted.*** Then we should create our own system. We damned sure could do a better job than those idiots in D.C.!!"

Without knowing it, the CEO was colorfully advocating *TexasCares*.

Third-party payment structure

Prior to 1930, there were only two *parties* in U.S. healthcare: *buyer* or patient, and *seller* as provider or hospital. There was no third party. Health insurance covered lost wages and paid a fixed amount to the patient after the patient paid the bill in full.

In the early 1930s, insurers began to offer insurance policies that were prepayment schemes for future health care needs. The patient paid a fixed amount monthly, and the insurer promised to pay any medical bills that arose. This is how insurance carriers became a *third party* to the transaction between buyer/patient and seller/provider.

Most people believe the rise of third-party payment systems occurred *in response* to the high cost of care. What few recognize is it was the opposite! The rise in the cost of care was caused by the development of third-party payment and the takeover of healthcare by Washington.

Third-party payment is not sustainable without medical rationing. Those who consume services and goods don't pay the bill. Those who provide care don't determine the price. A financing structure devoid of free market forces—buyers' incentive to economize and sellers' need to compete for buyers' dollars—is inherently unstable. Predictably, prices go up without limit, and shortages get worse. That is exactly what the public has experienced. Supply cannot balance demand. Because of instability and imbalance, complex insurance rules are passed as work-arounds or patches for a system that is not fiscally viable.

As the federal government created the rules for third-party payment, Washington gradually took over the entire healthcare system. The two root causes of healthcare system sickness are thus inextricably interwoven. First, federal control saps the lifeblood of healthcare: money. Second, federal rules protect a third-party payment structure that suppresses free market forces.

Federal control of healthcare and third-party payment is inconsistent with two founding principles of *TexasCares*: (1) It suppresses individual freedom. In fact, it returns us to a new form of an old tyranny, one we rejected nearly 250 years ago; (2) This deadly combination rejects personal responsibility. Now, the government is in charge and responsible, not you.

THAT is unacceptable to Texans and most Americans.

Incentives and Outcomes

To get an outcome you want, you need to give the right incentive to the right person, the one whose behavior determines the outcome.

When people talk about incentives, they often recite, "You catch more flies with honey than vinegar," or "Favor the carrot over the stick." It is true that positive incentives are much more effective that negative ones. It is better to offer a reward than threaten with punishment. But you have to choose the right incentive. Honey is good if you want to catch flies or influence people who like honey in their tea. (I don't, so honey would not be an effective incentive for me.) Carrots are good incentives for rabbits, just as tennis balls get Labrador Retrievers' undivided attention.

Incentives can be either *aligned* or *perverse.* Aligned means the behavior you reward will produce the outcome you desire. When you give your child a dollar for every "A" on the report card, you are likely to get lots of "A's." When you act perversely, see Figure 6-1.

A perverse incentive refers to one that encourages an outcome you *don't* want. I can hear you thinking, "Why would anyone do that?!"

Healthcare is rife with examples of perverse incentives. They are inherent in the third-party payment structure. The simplest might be the MCO (managed care organization) model. An MCO is paid an amount per member per month and gets to keep money they do not spend. That is their profit. Obviously, they have a very strong incentive *not* to spend money, which means *not* giving the care that people need. Obviously, this is a perverse incentive.

Figure 6-1: The Power of a Perverse Incentive

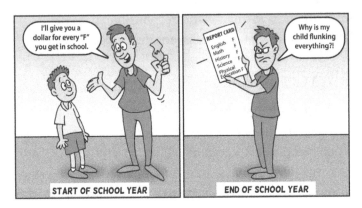

A second example are Pharmacy Benefits Management programs (PBM). Most health plans have PBMs and doctors in their network are required to use them. A doctor thinks a certain medication is the best one for you. To prescribe the medication, the doctor must first access the PBM on a computer. There, he sees a list of allowable medications that were selected primarily for low cost. Usually, the medication the doctor wants for the patient is not listed. So, he cannot prescribe what is not on the list. You get an inferior medicine, the cheapest one, chosen by a health plan bureaucrat, not your doctor.

Third-party payment incentives

Under the current third-party structure in healthcare, the buyers (patients) determine the demand for goods and services. Since they are spending OPM (other people's money), they have no incentive to economize. Their behavior is therefore to spend without restraint.

Insurance companies (the payers) have a powerful incentive not to pay for care, as that is how they generate profit. Their resulting behavior is the "three D" strategy: to defer, delay, and deny care because that is the best outcome for them: more profit. The outcome for patients is death-by-queueing.

In our current government-run, third-party payment system, bureaucrats make the insurance rules. What incentives do they have, how do they behave, and what is the outcome?

In today's healthcare system, providers of care have limited power to affect either patient outcomes, cost to their patients, or how much they themselves will be paid. Doctors do not decide what care patients get: insurance companies and federal mandates do. Providers have a very strong incentive to comply with federal regulations and hospital rules as their licenses to practice and their hospital privileges are at risk for noncompliance.

There is a way to change healthcare incentives from perverse to aligned: remove government control and stop third-party payment. We call that, *TexasCares*.

The Texas Model: *TexasCares*

What does healthcare look like without Washington and without a third-party payer? It is very simple. **Decision-making ability returns to the individual.** The system functions like buying a car.

Patient–as buyer and payer–is in charge

Say, you want to buy a new car. You look at your bank account and your income. You decide how much you can spend. Unlike the federal government, you can't spend more than you have.

You consider Ford, Honda, and Mercedes. You activate a car buying program on the internet and look up various models. You place them side by side on the screen. You compare price, maintenance costs, resale value, miles per gallon, and other features. You test drive the vehicles, decide which is the best value, and buy the car. You know you can afford the monthly payments because you first checked the cost compared to your monthly income and other obligations.

Now, switch focus to health care and *TexasCares*. You want a doctor for yourself or a pediatrician for your child, which means you want to purchase the care provider's services. You activate a medical shopping internet program and search for doctors within easy access. You refine your search based on factors such as price, wait times, years of experience, type of practice, satisfaction surveys, and even gender of the provider. You narrow down the list to three individuals and go visit them. (You are taking them for a test drive.)

You get a price list from the doctor for services you want or might need in the future. You check the funds in your *TexasCares* Health Savings Account (HSA). You decide which doctor is the best value and contract with that physician.

The government plays no role. It doesn't tell you what car to buy or which doctor to use. A federal bureaucrat doesn't say which automobile features or what insurance you must purchase. An insurance agent does not tell how long you will wait to get your car or your care. Even validation of miles per gallon and customer satisfaction surveys are done by independent, private companies.

Figure 6-2: TexasCares Is Simple

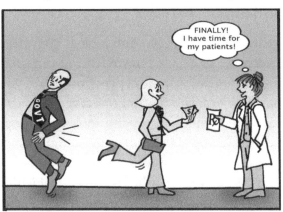

There is an important distinction between buying an automobile and purchasing health care. You don't *need* a high-priced Mercedes car. If you can't afford it, the lower-priced Honda or Ford will do just fine.

But when you have a heart attack, you need, really *need*, that very expensive operation and ICU stay. Nothing less will do. Without them, you will die. That is why you buy high-deductible insurance: to protect against financial catastrophe of the unexpected large medical bill—the auto accident or the surprise heart attack.

Many of the expensive and so-called unanticipated medical events can and should be anticipated. If a patient is a diabetic, the patient could shop in advance for the hospital to be taken to in the event of a collapse from too much or too little sugar in the blood. If a patient has a family history of heart disease, a high-stress job, weighs 350 pounds, and has a cholesterol level of 400, it would be prudent to discuss with his or her doctor where to go when the inevitable occurs. Plan in advance for the doctor and hospital you want!

High-priced, dramatic medical events like an auto crash, heart attack, or cancer, make eye-catching headlines and book titles, but a healthcare system should not be constructed primarily for the uncommon events.

Designing a healthcare system should start with the common events such as infections, rashes, diarrhea, sugar control in diabetics, asthma, blood pressure maintenance, delivering babies, arthritis, and minor trauma. The cash in HSAs will easily cover these expenses without any insurance involvement, especially with the lower prices produced by a market-based system. Big-ticket items like brain or heart surgery are where the high deductible insurance kicks in.

High deductible insurance in *TexasCares* would be quite different from what is currently available. With the policies you can buy today, insurance pays the provider an amount they decide in their contract with the provider, after you have paid the deductible. You can only use the doctor or hospital where the insurance company has a contract. You do not get to choose. You probably do not know how much the doctor is paid.

When you have *TexasCares* high deductible insurance, **you choose** the doctor. **You shop** for the best price, and **you pay** the bill. In the unusual circumstance where the bill exceeds the high deductible—for example, $5,000—the insurance policy might pay all of the unpaid balance over $5,000. You and the doctor agree in advance on the price. The insurance company has no part in determining how much the doctor receives—that is your decision.

Instead of the current win-lose scenario with its perverse incentives, *TexasCares* creates the win-win. With *TexasCares*, the patient seeks the best price and when he saves money, so does the insurance company. Incentives are now aligned.

For those enrolled in *TexasCares*, the combination of personal and state contributions into their HSAs along with high-deductible insurance provides a safety net.

However, *TexasCares* was not built exclusively for the Medicaid population. It was designed to be true to its founding principles, applicable to the general population, and then a safety net was added for the medically vulnerable.

TexasCares has three simple rules:

1. Money in an HSA can be used only for medical expenses.
2. Unused HSA funds can accumulate indefinitely.
3. Enrollees must purchase high-deductible health insurance of their choice.

"Medical expenses" are defined by the patient, not by the government or an insurance carrier. If a patient wants nontraditional medical care, such as acupuncture, crystal treatments, or aromatherapy, that is the patient's decision. As long as HSA funds are not used to buy cigarettes, alcohol, or a big-screen TV, in other words, as long as expenses are medical as the patient defines "medical," there are no restrictions on their use.

Money in HSAs

People enrolled in *TexasCares* will have "large HSAs," meaning well-funded, medical-use-only savings accounts. Enrollees shop for care and pay from the HSA on the day of service. Patients know the exact price they will pay and what services they will get. Doctors know what they will be paid, when, and what the patient expects.

Individuals spend their own money rather than other people's money (OPM). Thus, patients have some "skin in the game." At the same time, even in *TexasCares,* health care is expensive and beyond the pocket book of most Medicaid enrollees.

Enrollees in *TexasCares* put their own money into the HSA, say $500 per person, and the state matches that contribution with a larger amount. HSA funds are available for medical use by anyone in the family, or even a neighbor if the HSA holder chooses.

There is a time limit on state support for able-bodied adults. State contributions decline over a six-year period (see Table 6-1) and cease after six years. Texas expects nondisabled adults to become self-reliant by that time. For the disabled and the aged, matching contributions will continue indefinitely at the 18-to-1 level. Furthermore, contributions will continue for children at 8 to 1 until the child's 18th birthday.

	Multiplier		Family contribution	State contribution	Total HSA	Total HSA after expenses*
Year	Adult	Child				
1	18 to 1	8 to 1	$2,000	$26,000	$28,000	$13,000
2	18 to 1	8 to 1	$2,000	$26,000	$39,000	$24,000
3	14 to 1	8 to 1	$2,000	$22,000	$46,000	$31,000
4	14 to 1	8 to 1	$2,000	$22,000	$53,000	$38,000
5	10 to 1	8 to 1	$2,000	$18,000	$56,000	$41,000
6	10 to 1	8 to 1	$2,000	$18,000	$59,000	$44,000
7	0	0**	Optional	$0	$44,000	$27,000+
8	0	0**	Optional	$0	$12,000+	$12,000+

Table 6-1: HSA Funds Available Under TexasCares for Family of Four

Calculations are for a family of four, two adults and two children, assuming the family contributes $2,000 per year into their HSA. *TexasCares* insurance is assumed to cost $10,000 per year for the family. (*) Total family out-of-pocket expenses are $17,000: Insurance premium ($10,000) + spending on care up to deductible ($5000) + $2000 annual contribution to HSA. Compare to current average (non-Medicaid) family spending on healthcare of $28,166 in 2018. (**) It is possible one or more children will still be under age 19 years when the parents "time-out" of *TexasCares*. The state will continue to contribute 8 to 1 per child. For the calculations above, we did not consider these potential contributions. (+) The total HSA will be greater than shown above by the amount the family choses to contribute.

Individuals can contribute as much as they want, tax-free, at any time and the HSA remains with the family indefinitely, including if the primary account holder dies.

In 2018, Texas Medicaid will expend $30.6 billion on behalf of 4.1 million enrollees. That is $7,463 per person or $29,853 for a family of four. With *TexasCares*, the state will expend $22,500 for a family of four. That is only for the first two years. After that, the cost to the state declines as shown in Table 6-1.

One can also compare healthcare outlays in the non-Medicaid population for comparison with *TexasCares*. In 2018, the average American family will spend $28,166 on health insurance premiums, co-payments, and deductibles.[3] Imagine if that family could buy high deductible *TexasCares* insurance for $10,000 per year, put the remaining funds into their family HSA, and pay in cash for their general medical bills. Think how much they would have available to pay for care in just a few years.

Prices will plummet while payments will rise

Dramatic reduction in size of the healthcare bureaucracy will save Texas billions of dollars. The same is true in other states. Today, more than 40 percent of U.S. healthcare spending is consumed by the federal administrative bureaucracy, insurance companies, and regulatory compliance.[4] *TexasCares* cuts out these huge, wasteful costs. Doctors and hospitals will no longer have to pay, in both money and time, to comply with federal regulations and reviews. Those savings can be passed on to patients.

Second, there is the effect of market forces, well demonstrated in every endeavor where these natural forces are allowed to function freely, from energy production to buying a loaf of bread. The free market invariably gets the best products or services to the most people at the lowest prices. When a market is controlled by the government rather than by consumers, you see people shivering in the cold waiting in line for the government to distribute a limited supply of inferior but no-charge goods or services (Figure 6-3). In government-controlled healthcare, people die waiting in line for care.

Figure 6-3: Effects of a Centrally Controlled Economy

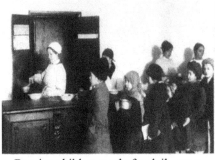 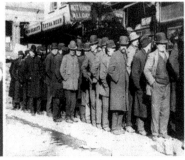

Russian children ready for daily soup   Russian men waiting in bread line

Some people have forgotten what the average person gets (or doesn't get) with central economic planning as in the now-defunct Union of Soviet Socialist Republics. Russians waited in line for hours to receive government handouts: soup or bread, a pair of "free" shoes with soles made from paper, or toilet paper that could also be used as sandpaper.

For those who think the U.S.S.R. is not a good analogy, note the shortages of doctors, operating rooms, and burn units in government-controlled healthcare systems in Canada and Great Britain.

Contrast government-controlled healthcare with concierge medicine in the U.S., also called direct-pay, no-insurance, or free market healthcare. Such practices avoid the hassle and the cost of insurance rules as well as federal administration and regulation. Direct-pay practices are like *TexasCares*: they directly connect buyer and seller—that's patient and doctor—with no third party in between.

Data from direct-pay practices show that prices go down and payments go up. In Table 6-2, you note that Medicaid pays 22 percent to 54 percent of the doctor's charges. The billed charges of the direct-pay practice are consistently *lower* than insurance, and yet, the doctor gets paid more in every instance. Elimination of third-party, government involvement produces better and cheaper care at the same time.

Table 6-2: Direct Pay versus Government Insurance				
	Average Total Charges		Average Total Payment	
Procedure	Univ. Hosp.	SCO	SCO	Medicaid
Childbirth, vaginal	$4,719	$3,111	$3,111	$2,557
Cataract surgery, one eye	$7,390	$4,000	$4,000	$1,637
Laparoscopic repair, inguinal hernia, one side	$12,043	$5,750	$5,750	$3,157
Hip replacement, one side	$35,114	$15,499	$15,499	$12,922
Univ. Hosp.=University of New Mexico Health Sciences Center. SCO=Surgery Center of Oklahoma, Oklahoma City, OK, a direct-pay, no-insurance medical facility.				

Personal responsibility and welfare roles

Ronald Reagan began welfare reform in California in the 1970's as Governor and carried that forward nationally in the 1980s as president. He is frequently quoted as saying, "We should measure welfare's success by how many people leave welfare, not by how many are added." In today's world of entitlements, we should add, "nor should we measure success by how much the government gives those on welfare."

Figure 6-4: What Welfare Should Be Instead of What It Is

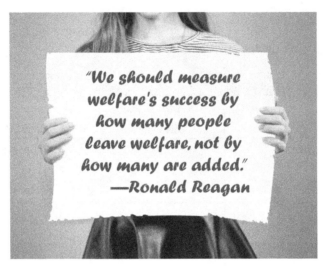

"We should measure welfare's success by how many people leave welfare, not by how many are added."
—Ronald Reagan

In the U.S., where people pride themselves on resourcefulness, ingenuity, and self-reliance, welfare should be *temporary* assistance until the recipient of government charity gets back on his or her feet. Welfare should be a short-term helping hand while someone goes from dependence on other people's money given by the state to independence, the natural condition of Americans.

It is clearly understood that an expectation of independence, and therefore only temporary government aid, does not apply to those who might never be independent: aged, blind, disabled, or genetic disorders.

In 1996, under Democrat President Bill Clinton and a Republican-led Congress, PRWORA (Personality Responsibility and Work Opportunity Reconciliation Act) was passed. It was a fundamental cultural shift for welfare, changing from an entitlement to personal responsibility.

The programs altered in 1996 were Supplemental Nutritional Assistance Program (SNAP) or food stamps, and Temporary

Assistance for Needy Families (TANF), which had previously been called Aid to Families with Dependent Children. SNAP provided food and TANF gave cash. Both imposed requirements on the recipients such as co-payments, time limits for support (after all, it is "temporary"), and job training or job seeking. The recipient received a government contribution in return for performing one or more of these "work requirements."

Even before passage of PRWORA, nanny-state advocates were predicting doomsday. People would starve to death, no one would get jobs, incomes would go down, and millions of children would be driven into poverty or foster care. The exact opposite happened.

In 2006, ten years after PRWORA was passed, the results were assessed and reported to Congress.[5] After conversion of entitlements to programs with personal responsibility, welfare recipients got good-paying jobs, no one starved, children were better off, and the numbers on welfare dropped.

Similar positive results are likely to result from *TexasCares*, which by design, has personal responsibility built in. Not only will Medicaid roles decline, but people who are personally responsible are healthier. Ask any family physician or general physician. Persons who accept personal responsibility take better care of themselves instead of waiting for the government to take care of them.

I learned a wonderful phrase in a meeting with a hard-core-capitalist-turned-philanthropist. He was setting up free medical clinics in Texas and demanded that people coming for care pay a small amount upon entrance to the clinic. Some might call this a co-payment but technically that would be wrong as there is no insurance *co*-payer. The CEO called this a "dignity payment," a way to recognize the patient as an adult, responsible individual who can hold his head up high—with dignity. I like that, a lot.

Effect on state budget

For fiscal year 2018, Texas is slated to spend $30.6 billion on its Medicaid program. Assuming a similar dollar efficiency in the Lone Star State as national, 60 percent of its spending,[4] or $18,360,000,000, will pay for health care in any form.

The cost of *TexasCares* for the year 2018 was calculated at $26.5 billion. The role and therefore the cost of bureaucracy is quite small, certainly less than 5 percent. As *TexasCares* will be at least 95 percent dollar efficient, $25,175,000,000 will go to pay for care. Thus, with no increase in state spending, $6,815,000,000 additional dollars will become available to pay for care.

In plain English, *TexasCares* is a win-win-win scenario. It is affordable for patients who get the care they need, care providers are paid more, and it is cheaper for the state. Pretty good deal for all Americans, except federal bureaucrats and politicians—who lose the control they crave.

Texas model for general population?

TexasCares can satisfy the medical needs of the Medicaid population. What about the majority of Americans, those who do not qualify for state support? Would the Texas model work for them too?

The answer is yes! As noted previously, in 2018 the average American family will expend $28,166 for health insurance premiums, co-pays, and deductibles. That amount is 48 percent of the family's total income. Imagine if the family could put $28,166 into an HSA every year, purchase high-deductible insurance, such as a $5,000 deductible, and pay for their own care from an HSA. Imagine how much money, and independence, they would have!

With the Texas model, the family would pay for insurance out of the HSA and not need employer-supported insurance. Employer expenditures for health insurance could then be given to the employee as compensation. The market would no longer be distorted by the tax preference of employer-supported insurance. As an added benefit, insurance would be truly portable, not tied to one's employment.

Finally, the majority of Americans would be free to make their own care decisions instead of having an insurance agent or a federal bureaucrat decide *for* them. That would be a most welcome change.

So, yes, the Texas model—*TexasCares*—would work very well for all Americans, not only for the Medicaid population in Texas.

That's it!

TexasCares is simple and easy to use. Here is a list of healthcare activities **_NOT_** present in *TexasCares*:

- pre-authorization process
- eligibility forms
- verification procedure
- approval/disapproval of care decisions
- advanced premium tax credits
- market stabilization payments (subsidies) to insurance companies
- delay of care
- denial of care
- limited list of available doctors
- long wait times (queueing)
- pre-determined payment (reimbursement) schedule
- discount-from-charges
- billing and coding

- o regulatory compliance
- o multiple reviews
- o accountants, actuaries, administrators, agents, billers and coders, bureaucrats, compliance officers, consultants, in-person assisters, lawyers, middlemen, navigators, regulators, reviewers, rule writers
- o all the costs in money and time associated with federal control and third-party payments

"Elevator pitch" for TexasCares

Management experts challenge someone who has a new idea to pitch or sell it in the time it takes an elevator to go to the tenth floor, i.e., less than a minute. This is called the "elevator pitch." Here is my elevator pitch for *TexasCares*, in 60 words, or about 25 seconds.

With TexasCares, the patient chooses the caregiver, decides the care, agrees to the price, pays the bill, and evaluates the result. Insurance carriers and care providers compete for the patient's business. Neither government nor insurance has any say in your medical decisions. TexasCares offers the best balance of free market dollar efficiency with society's need to protect the medically vulnerable.

Chapter Notes

1. Of course, I am referring to the Tenth Amendment to the U.S. Constitution, "The powers not delegated to the United States by the Constitution, nor prohibited by it to the States, are reserved to the States respectively, or to the people."
2. I have authored numerous articles proposing and explaining *StatesCare* as well as *TexasCares* in venues

such as *Fox News, The Hill, Washington Examiner, NewzGroup, The Daily Caller,* and *RealClear Health.* I may or may not be the first, but I claim to be the loudest.

3. Milliman Medical Index projects the average U.S. family of four will spend more than $28,166 in total healthcare expenses in 2018.

4. Minimum estimates of the cost of the healthcare bureaucracy are 31 percent and 40 percent. Both estimates were made before the implementation of the Affordable Care Act, with its $2 trillion administrative price tag.

5. On July 19, 2006, Ron Haskins testified before Congress on his compilation of all the evidence of effect resulting from implementation of PRWORA. He gave a detailed, balanced, and completely non-partisan presentation.

Chapter 7:

Questions & Answers

A new healthcare system is bound to raise concerns. Here are questions (Q, in bold) that I have been asked followed by my best answers (A).

Q: **Isn't your *TexasCares* HSA just like what is now called an FSA?**

A: "FSA" stands for flexible savings account, which is a medical-use only bank account in which employees and sometimes employers contribute pre-tax dollars. Unlike the HSAs in *TexasCares*, today's FSA has an upper limit for contributions; you must use-it-or-lose-it within one year; and the employer, not the patient, defines what is "medical use."

Q: **With your free market, profit-driven *TexasCares* plan, won't poor people be left to die in the streets?**

A₁: In *TexasCares*, poor people will be covered by the safety net with large HSAs and high deductible insurance. Providers will readily accept them into their medical or surgical practices because they are cash patients. They won't be dying in the streets.

A₂: Second, the people today who are "dying in the streets" generally have government insurance. Earlier in this book

I described Americans experiencing death-by-queueing in Illinois, Maryland, and the VA system.[1]

A₃: The main beneficiary of profit in *TexasCares* are the patients, followed closely by the providers. Patients get control of their money and will be able to spend less. Doctors whose patients do well will be rewarded with profit. Even insurance companies will profit; however, with *TexasCares*, insurance companies profit when patients do well and not when carriers deny or delay care.

Q: What happens when enrollees run out of money?

A₁: In *TexasCares*, disabled, aged, and children will never run out of money because the state will continue its support indefinitely, as it does now. For able-bodied adults, state support ceases after six years and at that time, they are responsible for themselves and should be self-reliant.

A₂: If the Texas model were adopted for the whole state, some of the 25 million Texans who are not eligible for Medicaid might choose to contribute insufficient funds into their HSAs or not contribute at all and not purchase insurance. They would then be responsible for their medical bills. If necessary, they would file for bankruptcy. The freedom to make choices comes with the obligation to accept the consequences.

Q: Would doctors and hospitals willingly compete with each other? They certainly won't want to. Don't we need the government to force them to compete?

A₁: Keep in mind that government mandates in healthcare got us into this mess in the first place. No, we don't want or need federal or state government to enforce competition. The market will take care of those who refuse to give shoppers the information they need.

A$_2$: If a doctor or hospital refuses to provide the necessary data up front or provides confusing information, you know what will happen: consumers, spending their own money as they see fit, won't buy from the sellers who do not provide data they need in a form they can use. Will doctors willingly compete? Only the ones who want to stay in business. For my medical colleagues, don't forget that in a market-based system such as direct-pay where government controls are absent, doctors will make more money, not less.

Q: **Will *TexasCares* work for the general, non-Medicaid population?**

A: *TexasCares* was designed on principles, not for a specific population. It will work for Medicaid enrollees. It will work for the other 25 million Texans. If other states want to emulate the Texas model, it will work elsewhere too, but only if the other states' residents want *TexasCares*. No system should be imposed on them.

Q: **If your idea is so good and obvious, why has no one done it before?**

A: Government is always the one "fixing" healthcare. Yet government is the root cause of the problem. So, every fix they enact makes healthcare worse, not better. People are starting free market medical and surgical practices with no government involvement and enjoying great success for both doctors and patients. In Texas, four <u>Free Market Surgery</u> centers have recently opened.

Q: **What happens to CHIP under *TexasCares*?**

A: The Children's Health Insurance Program (CHIP) is a jointly funded, state–federal program to provide health insurance coverage for children in impoverished families whose incomes are above the threshold for Medicaid and less than 200 percent to 300 percent of federal poverty level, depending on the state.

CHIP is different from Medicaid with respect to eligibility. Washington's CHIP contributions to states are higher than for Medicaid. CHIP has an element of personal responsibility—cost-sharing by the family—that is not present in Medicaid. CHIP is less expensive than Medicaid—$156 per child per month—while Medicaid costs $237 per child per month. In 2016, 352,432 children were enrolled in Texas CHIP.

With *TexasCares,* the state of Texas will determine eligibility for enrollment. If the standards chosen **do not** include the children currently in CHIP, then there will be no change in that program. If the new standards **do** include the children currently in CHIP, then they will be folded into *TexasCares* and the amount of the block grant will need to be adjusted upwards to compensate.

Q: What kind of preparation would be needed if *TexasCares* goes forward?

A: First, a global waiver of all federal mandates and a fixed-sum block grant, will be negotiated between Austin and Washington. Then well in advance of a start date, there will be an extensive informational campaign presented to sellers—doctors, therapists, hospitals, pharmacies, insurance carriers, etc.—about what the consumers will expect from them, and to consumers about what their choices and responsibilities are. This is not a mandate in any way but merely advisory. The only mandates in *TexasCares* are the following: buyers (patients) must use their HSAs for medical costs only, and they must purchase high deductible insurance. For sellers, one mandate might be a penalty for false advertising. That would be up to the state of Texas.

Q: **Won't this be too big a shock to the country and the people?**

A: The Texas model certainly will be a big change for everyone. Doctors and insurers would suddenly have to function in a free market setting, which they have not done for more than eighty years. For consumers, it would be a smaller change as they now function in a free market for everything, except healthcare and education. For federal legislators, *StatesCare* would be a bitter pill: they would have to cede power (control) to the states. For state legislators, the freedom from Washington will be both scary and invigorating.

All shocks can be scary: *different* is always frightening. Not all shocks are bad. If you get a big raise in your paycheck, you are excited and happy, yet scared that you won't get another one next year.

Q: **How can you be so sure that *TexasCares* will drive costs down?**

A: It will drive costs down because *TexasCares* makes sense in theory and has been proven in practice. Economics 101 teaches us that free market forces produce the best balance of supply and demand, that you get the most product or service of the highest quality for the best price when buyers spend their own money and sellers compete for buyers' dollars. Look at the history of cell phones or Lasik surgery as examples of what happens when a product or service is exposed to free market forces.

Q: **We all know, "if it sounds too good to be true, it _is_!" Can you really get both better and cheaper health care?**

A: This aphorism has been proven time again, yet I stand by my assertion. Better and cheaper are possible in healthcare. With central economic planning, i.e., government control of healthcare, you can have *either* better *or* cheaper, but *never both*. BOTH are available in a free market. Whether you are buying a car, having Lasik surgery, or getting a divorce online, both better and cheaper can be found when sellers compete and buyers economize.

Q: **Won't *TexasCares* put a lot of people, possibly millions, out of work?**

A: Yes, it will. The people who become unnecessary are healthcare administrators, bureaucrats, consultants, and lawyers whose salaries and benefits you have been paying for decades. Don't you want to stop wasting your "healthcare" dollars on them and spend your money on yourself?

Q: **Why has the cost of healthcare in the U.S. become so completely unaffordable?**

A_1: There are two reasons: one is value and the other is a waste.

A_2: My grandfather graduated from the University of Pennsylvania Medical School in 1913. In his time, there were no clot-busting drugs; no heart surgery; no cures for any form of cancer; or patients with "known" complex congenital heart diseases. So, people with blood clots in their lungs, heart attacks, cancer, or my babies (pediatric cardiology patients) with holes in their hearts, they all died. Medical care was very cheap because doctors couldn't do much. There was very limited value available for the healthcare dollar because there was very little technology.

All the conditions mentioned above can now be treated. These treatments are expensive to create, to get FDA approval, to produce, and to use. They are costly but valuable to patients because they save the lives of people who would otherwise die.

In 1960, before all the massive technological advances we enjoy today, the U.S. spent $147 per person on healthcare. In 2018, we will spend $10,526. That is a 7,161 percent increase in healthcare spending. Over the same period, net inflation was 727 percent for other spending.

A_3: In my grandfather's day, there was no insurance as prepayment and no federal healthcare bureaucracy to speak of. The costs associated with third-party payment and government bureaucracy—now approaching half of all healthcare spending—simply did not exist.

Q: **Healthcare is too complex for people to understand. They need guidance.**

A_1:   The current system IS too complex. And that complexity is unnecessary. The *TexasCares* system is quite simple and works just like shopping for other goods or services, something people do every day.

A_2: "Guidance" is code for control.[2] Americans can either control themselves and be free, or they can accept government control and be dependent. There really is no in between.

Chapter Notes

1. Illinois expanded its Medicaid program under Obamacare. As a result, many more people were insured. Sounds like a good outcome, but wait. ... After paying the insurance companies for the mandated benefits, there was too little money left over to pay the providers. Just like New Mexico, Illinois had to reduce its already low reimbursement schedule to doctors even further. This meant fewer providers would accept these low government

payment schedules. The effect was to increase insurance coverage and decrease access to care. Bottom line, as reported by Nicholas Horton, "752 Illinoisans on the state's Medicaid waiting list have died awaiting needed care."

○ The story of the needless death of a 12-year old boy in Maryland, Deamonte Driver, was described in Chapter 1.

○ In 2015, the VA health system, our home-grown American single payer system, performed an <u>audit</u> to determine if veterans were receiving the medial care they needed. The auditors concluded that, "307,000 veterans may have died" while waiting for approval to receive care.

○ The consequence of Medicaid expansion is proven: enrollment increases, cost of insurance coverage goes up, further cuts to payments to providers, and so, as enrollment increases, access to care decreases. What I fail to comprehend is why people claim expansion is a good thing, and why some many states keep their expansion programs.

2. Every advisory, algorithm, counsel, direction, guideline, one-pager, opinion, and recommendation coming out of Washington has been turned into enforceable commandments by hospital risk management departments. The very last thing that healthcare needs, or more accurately, the last thing that *patients* need, is "guidance" from Washington.

Author's Evidence (References)

AAFP (American Academy of Family Physicians). 2018. "Direct Primary Care."

Ackoff RL, Emery FE. 1972. On Purposeful Systems. Chicago: Aldine-Atherton.

Ackoff RL. 1978. The Art of Problem Solving, Accompanied by Ackoff's Fables. Wiley & Sons, New York.

Ackoff RL. 1989. From Data to Wisdom. *Journal of Applied Systems Analysis* 16: 3-9.

Ackoff RL. 1999. Ackoff's Best: His Classic Writings on Management. Wiley & Sons, New York.

Ackoff RL, Rovin S. 2003. Redesigning Society. Stanford Business Books: Stanford, C.

ADHS (Arkansas Department of Human Services). 2018. "Arkansas Works."

Aiken LH, Clarke SP, Sloane DM, et al., October 23/30, 2002. Hospital Nurse Staffing and Patient Mortality, Nurse Burnout, and Job Dissatisfaction. *Journal of the American Medical Association,* 286(16): 1987-1993.

Alexander JA, Fennell M. 1986. Patterns of decision making in multihospital systems. *Journal of Health and Social Behavior,* 27(1): 14-27.

Alexander JA, Lichtenstein R, Oh H, Ullman E. 1998. A causal model of voluntary turnover among nursing personnel in long-term psychiatric settings. *Research in Nursing and Health* 21(5): 415-427.

Allen SW, Gauvreau K, Bloom BT, Jenkins KJ. 2003. Evidence-based referral results in significantly reduced mortality after congenital heart surgery. *Pediatrics* 112(1): 24-28.

Amadeo, Kimberly. 2017. "How much did Obamacare cost?" *The Balance.*

Anderson GF, Hussey PS, Frogner BK, Waters HR. 2005. Health spending in the United States and the rest of the industrialized world. *Health Affairs* 24(4): 903-914.

Angell M. 10/13/02. Forgotten domestic crisis. *New York Times,* Op-Ed.

Anonymous. Mar/Apr 2003. Research Notes. *Healthcare Executive* 18(2): 42.

Anonymous. Jul/Aug 2004. Hospital CEO turnover remains stable in 2003. *Healthcare Executive* 19(4): 65.

Antonisse, Larisa, and Rachel Garfield. 2018. *The Relationship Between Work and Health: Findings from a Literature Review.* Kaiser Family Foundation.

AP News. August 2018. "Lawsuit filed over Arkansas Medicaid work requirement."

"America's Health Future." May 2018. Interview with CMS Administrator Seema Verma et al. *Washington Post.*

Argote L, Epple D. 1990. Learning Curves in Manufacturing. *Science,* Feb 247: 920–24.

Argüellos, JR de P. 2008. Welfare rights and health care. In: Weisstub DN, Diaz Pintos G. 2008. Autonomy and Human Rights in Health Care. Springer: The Netherlands.

Aronson D. 1996-98. Overview of Systems Thinking. www.thinking.net. Accessed Feb 2004.

Arndt M, Bigelow B. 2000. The transfer of business practices into hospitals: history and implications. *Advances in Health Care Management* Vol. 1: 339-368.

Ashkanasy NM, Broadfoot LE, Falkus S. 2000. Questionnaire measures of organizational culture. In Neal M. Ashkanazy,

Celeste P. M. Wilderon, and Mark F. Peterson (Eds.), Handbook of organizational culture and climate (pp. 131-145). Thousand Oaks, CA: Sage Publications.

Ashmos DP, McDaniel RR. 1991. Physician participation in hospital strategic decision making: The effect of hospital strategy and decision content. *Health Services Research* 26(3): 375-401.

Ashmos DP, McDaniel RR. 1996. Understanding the participation of critical task specialists in strategic decision making. *Decision Science* Winter 27(1): 103-121.

Ashmos DP, Duchon D, McDaniel RR. 1998. Participation in strategic decision making: The role of organizational predisposition and issue interpretation. *Decision Science* 29(1): 25-51.

Ashmos DP, Huonker JW, McDaniel RR. 1998. The effect of clinical professional and middle manager participation on hospital performance. *Health Care Management Review* 23(4): 7-20.

Ashmos DP, Duchon D, McDaniel RR. 2000. Organizational response to complexity: the effect on organizational performance. *Journal of Organizational Change* 13(6): 577-594.

Associated Press, April 4, 2007. Doctor contrasts his cancer care with uninsured patient who died. Accessed March 2009 at: www.cnn.com/2007/HEALTH/04/04/uninsured.dead.ap/index.html.

Associated Press. April 18, 2007. Researchers: Let's Scrap the Internet and Start Over. Accessed May 14, 2007 at: www.foxnews.com/story/0,2933,266124,00.html.

Atwater JB, Pittman PH. 2006. Facilitating systemic thinking in business classes. *Decision Sciences Journal of Innovative Education*, July, 4(2): 273-292.

Axelsson R. 1998. Toward an evidence-based health care management. *International Journal of Health Planning and Management* 13; 307-17.

Baiker K, Taubman SL, Allen HL, et al. 2013. The Oregon Experiment—Effects of Medicaid on clinical outcomes. *New England Journal of Medicine,* 368;18: 1713-22.

Baker E. 2001. Learning from the Bristol Inquiry. *Cardiology in the Young* 11: 585-587.

Baker T. 1999. Doing Well by Doing Good, Economic Policy Institute, Washington, DC.

Baloff, N. 1971. Extension of the Learning Curve—Some Empirical Results. *Operational Research Quarterly* 1971; 22(4): 329–40.

Barnard A, Tong K. 2000. The doctor is out. *Boston Globe*, July 9: A18.

Barzansky B, Etzel SI. September 5, 2001. Educational programs in the US medical schools 2000-2001. *Journal of American Medical Association* 286(9): 1049-1055

Bass CD. 2000. Medicine losing its workhorses. *Albuquerque Journal*, September 17, 2000; page I-2.

Barrett R. January 27, 2002. The Apprentices--Construction trades need more people willing to learn while they earn. *Albuquerque Journal* I-1 & 2.

Barron JM, McCafferty S. September 1977. Job search, labor supply, and the quit decision: Theory and evidence. *American Economic Review* 67(4): 683-691.

Bartol KM. December 1979. Professionalism as a predictor of organizational commitment, role stress, and turnover: A multidimensional approach. *Academy of Management Journal* 22(4): 815-821.

Bates DW, Boyle DL, Vander Vliet MB, et al. 1995. Relationship between medication errors and adverse drug events. *Journal of General Internal Medicine* 10(4) 199-205, DOI: 10.1007/BFO2600255.

BCCS (Breast and Cervical Cancer Support) Eligibility. *Texas Health and Human Services.* Accessed August 2018.

Becker T. 2004. Why pragmatism is not practical. *Journal of Management Inquiry September* 13(3): 224-230. See Jacobs (2004) for companion article.

Beedham T. 1996. Why do young doctors leave medicine? *British Journal of Hospital Medicine* 55(11): 699-701. Editorial Comments by Elizabeth Paice 1997; 90(8): 417-418 and by John Davis 1997; 90(10): 585.

Begg CB, Cramer LD, Hoskins WJ, Brennan MF. 1998. Impact of Hospital Volume on Operative Mortality for Cancer Surgery. *Journal of the American Medical Association* 280: 1747–51.

Beinhocker, ED. 1997. Strategy at the edge of chaos. *The McKinsey Quarterly* Winter #1, pp. 24-40.

Beller GA. 2000. Academic Health Centers: The making of a crisis and potential remedies. *Journal of the American College of Cardiology* 36:1428-31.

Bender C, DeVogel S, Blomberg R. 1999. The socialization of newly hired medical staff into a large health system. *Health Care Management Review* 24:95-108.

Berenson RA Ginsburg PB, May JH. 2007. Hospital-physician relations: Cooperation, competition, or separation? *Health Affairs* 26(1): w31-w43.

Berger JE, Boyle RL. November/December 1992. How to avoid the high costs of physician turnover. *MGM Journal* pp. 80-91.

Berry LL. 2004. The Collaborative Organization: Leadership lessons from Mayo Clinic. *Organizational Dynamics* 33(3): 228-242.

Berta WB, Baker R. 2004. Factors that impact the transfer and retention of best practices for reducing error in hospital. *Health Care Management Review* 29(2): 90-97.

(von) Bertalanffy L. 1968. General System theory: Foundation, development, applications. George Braziller, New York, revised edition 1976.

Berwick DM. 1989. Continuous Improvement as an ideal in health care. *New England Journal of Medicine* 320(1): 53-56.

Berwick DM, Godfrey AB, Roessner J. 1990. Curing Health Care. Jossey-Bass, San Francisco, CA.

Betlach, Thomas J. April 2, 2018. Thomas J. Betlach to Douglas A. Ducey, Steve Yarbrough, and J.D. Mesnard. Arizona Health Care Cost Containment System.

Bettis RW, Prahahald CK. 1995. The dominant logic: retrospective and extension. *Strategic Management Journal* 16(1): 237-252.

Beyer JM, Trice HM: "Using Six Organizational Rites to Change Culture" pages 370-399. In: Kilmann RH, Saxton MJ, Serpa R, et al (1985) Gaining Control of the Corporate Culture. San Francisco: Jossey-Bass.

Birkmeyer JD, Finlayson SR, Tosteson AN, et al. 1999. "Effect of Hospital Volume on In-hospital Mortality with Pancreaticoduodenectomy." *Surgery* 125: 250–56

Birkmeyer JD, Stukel TA, Siewers AE, et al. 2003. Surgeon volume and operative mortality in the United States. *New England Journal of Medicine* 349: 2117-27.

Bisognano M. 2004. What Juran says. One of four essays on "Can the gurus' concepts cure healthcare?" In *Quality Progress* September pp. 33-34.

Blackburn R, Rosen B. 1993. Total quality and human resource management: lessons learned from Baldrige award-winning companies. *Academy of Management Executive* 7: 49-66.

Blaufuss J, Maynard J, Schollars G. 1992a. Calculating and Updating Nursing Turnover Costs. *Nursing Economic$* January/February 10(1): 39-45, 78.

Blaufuss J, Maynard J, Schollars G. 1992b. Methods of evaluating turnover costs. *Nursing Management* 23(5): 52-59.

Blahous, Charles. July 30, 2018. The Costs of National Single-Payer Healthcare System. Mercatus Center, George Mason University.

Bloom J, Alexander JA, Nuchols B. 1992. The effect of the social organization of work on the voluntary turnover rate of hospital nurses in the United States. *Social Science and Medicine* 34(12): 1413-1424.

Blumenthal D, Hsiao. September 15, 2005. Privatization and Its Discontents-The Evolving Chinese Health Care System. *New England Journal of Medicine* 353: 1165-1170.

Bole TJ, Bondeson W. 1991. Rights to Health Care. Kluwer Academic Publishers: London.

Bolster CJ, Hawthorne G, Schubert P. Nov/Dec 2002. Executive compensation survey: Can money buy happiness? *Trustee* 55(10): 8-12.

Bonacich, P. 1987. Power and Centrality: A Family of Measures. *American Journal of Sociology* 92(5): 1170-82.

Borda RG, Norman IJ. 1997. Factors influencing turnover and absence of nurses: a research review. *International Journal of Nursing Studies* 34(6): 385-394.

Bowles S, Gintis H. 1998. The Evolution of Strong Reciprocity. Santa Fe Institute Working Paper, SFI 98-08-073E. Accessed on January 14, 2007 at: http://citeseer.ist.psu.edu/bowles98evolution.html.

Boyd, Dan. March 5, 2016. NM faces $417M Medicaid shortfall. *Albuquerque Journal*.

Bradbury, R. 1966. Farenheit 451. Sundance Books, Littleton, MA. Reprinted 2002.

Bragg JE, Andrews IR. 1973. Participative decision-making: An experimental study in a hospital. *Journal of Applied Behavioral Science* 9: 727-735.

Brass DJ. 1984. Being in the right place: A structural analysis of individual influence in an organization. *Administrative Science Quarterly*, 29: 518-539.

Brass DJ, Burkhardt ME. 1993. Potential power and power use: An investigation of structure and behavior. *Academy of Management Journal* 36(3): 441-470.

Brennan TA, Localio AR, Leape LL, et al. 1990. Identification of Adverse Effects Occurring during Hospitalization: A Cross-Sectional Study of Litigation, Quality Assurance, and Medical Records at Two Teaching Hospitals. *Annals of Internal Medicine* 112: 221-226.

Brennan TA, Sox CM, Burstin HR. 1996. Relation Between Negligent Adverse Events and the Outcomes of Medical-Malpractice Litigation. *New England Journal of Medicine* 335:1963-1967.

Brewer LA, Fosburg RG, Mulder GA, Verska JJ (1972) Spinal cord complications following surgery for coarctation of the aorta. *Journal of Thoracic and Cardiovascular Surgery* 64(3): 368-381.

Brook RH, Lohr KN (1987) Monitoring quality of care in the Medicare Program. *Journal of the American Medical Association* 258: 3138-3141.

Bristol Royal Infirmary Inquiry Final Report, July 2001; Accessed March 15, 2006 at: www.bristol-inquiry.org.uk/final_report/index.htm.

Brockschmidt, FR. 1996. Corporate culture: does it play a role in health care management? *Certified Registered Nurse Anesthetist* 1994; 5:93-6.

Broder DS. October 21, 2001. Need for capable government has never been clearer. *Albuquerque Journal,* B2.

Broder DS. April 17, 2002. Health cost spike can't be ignored. *Albuquerque Journal,* A12.

Broder DS. March 18, 2005. Unfunded mandates still plaguing states, cities. *Albuquerque Journal*, #77, A14.

Brooks I. 1996. Using rituals to reduce barriers between sub-cultures. *Journal of Management in Medicine* 10(3): 23-30.

Brotherton SE, Simon FA, Etzel SI (September 5, 2001) US Graduate medical education 2000-2001. *Journal of American Medical Association* 286(9): 1056-1060.

Bruner EM, Ed. 1983. Text, play, and story: the construction and reconstruction of self and society: 1983 Proceedings of the American Ethnological Society. Waveland Press; Prospect Heights, Ill, 1988.

Bryan-Brown C, Dracup K. 2001. An Essay on Criticism. *American Journal of Critical Care* 10(1): 1-4

Bryson RW, Aderman M, Sampiere JM, Rockmore L, Matsuda T. 1985. Intensive care nurse: Job tension and satisfaction as a function of experience level. *Critical Care Medicine* 13(9): 767-769.

Buchan J, Seccombe I. June 13, 1991. The high cost of turnover. *Health Services Journal* 101(5256): 27-28.

Buckbinder SB, Wilson M, Melick CF, Powe NR. 2001. Primary care physician job satisfaction and turnover. *American Journal of Managed Care* 7(7): 701-713.

Buckingham M, Coffman C. 1999. First, Break All The Rules. Simon and Schuster: New York

Burne J. April 16, 2005. Cleaning up MRSA. *The [London] Times*, A12.

Burt RS, MJ Miner MJ (eds.) 1983. Applied Network Analysis: A Methodological Introduction. Beverly Hills: Sage.

Bush, H, et al. Abstract 881. Presented at: Digestive Disease Week; June 2-5, 2018; Washington, D.C

Butterworth P., et al. 2011. "The psychosocial quality of work determines whether employment has benefits for mental health: results from a longitudinal national household panel survey." *Occupational and Environmental Medicine* 68(11): 806-812.

California Healthline, March 20, 2009. Suit Says Lab Firms Overbilled Medi-Cal for Testing Services. Accessed April 2009 at: http://www.californiahealthline.org/Articles/2009/3/20/ Suit-Says-Lab-Firms-Overbilled-MediCal-for-Testing-Services.aspx.

Cameron KS, Freeman SJ. 1991. Cultural congruence, Strength, and Type: Relationships to Effectiveness. *Research in Organizational Change and Development* 5: 23-58.

Carleson, Susan A. 2012. The Reagan Remedy for Medicaid. *AmericanThinker.com*

Carroll L. Reprinted in 1994. Alice in Wonderland and Through the Looking-Glass. Quality Paperback Book Club: New York.

Cassata D. AP, May 8, 2011. Health care costs a hefty price tag for Pentagon. Accessed May 8, 2011 at: http://www.wtop.com/?nid=209&sid=2374508.

Carvel J. November 23, 2005. NHS cash crisis bars knee and hip replacements for obese. *Manchester Guardian*, Page 1.

93a. Catron D. April 15, 2013. The Wheels Come Off Obamacare. *American Spectator* at: http://spectator.org/archives/2013/04/15/the-wheels-come-off-obamacare.

Cavanaugh SJ. 1990. Predictors of Nursing staff turnover. *Journal of Advanced Nursing* 15(3): 373-380.

Champy J. 1995. Reengineering Management. HarperBusiness: New York.

Charles SC, Gibbons RD, Frisch PR, et al. 1992. Predicting Risk for Medical Malpractice Claims Using Quality-of-Care Characteristics. *Western Journal of Medicine* 157:433-439.

Chassin MR. 1998. Is health care ready for six sigma quality? *The Millbank Quarterly* Winter v76 i4 p 565(2).

Christenson CM, Bohmer R, Kenagy J. 2000. Will disruptive innovations cure health care? *Harvard Business Review* 78(5): 102-112.

Clark RE. 1996. Outcome as a Function of Annual Coronary Artery Bypass Graft Volume. *Annals of Thoracic Surgery* 6(1): 21–26.

Claybrook J. 2004. Don't blame lawsuits for rising malpractice insurance rates. *USA Today* Tuesday January 27; p. 19A.

Clinton, William J. August 22, 1996. "Statement on Signing the Personal Responsibility and Work Opportunity Reconciliation Act of 1996." *The American Presidency Project.*

Cochrane AL. 1972. Effectiveness and Efficiency: Random Reflections of Health Services. London: Nuffield Trust.

Coeling HVE, Wilcox JR. 1988. Understanding organizational culture: A key to management decision-making. *Journal of Nursing Administration* 18(11): 16-24.

Coeling HVE, Simms LM. 1993. Facilitating Innovations at the Nursing Unit Level through Cultural Assessment, Part 1: How to keep Management Ideas from Falling on Deaf Ears. *Journal of Nursing Administration* 23: 46-53.

Coeling HVE, Simms LM. 1993. Facilitating Innovation at the unit level through cultural assessment, Part 2. *Journal of Nursing Administration* 23(5): 13-20.

Cohn KH, Peetz ME. 2003. Surgeon frustration: Contemporary problems, practical solutions. *Contemporary Surgery.* 59(2): 76-85.

Cohn KH, Gill S, Schwartz R. 2005. Gaining hospital administrators' attention: Ways to improve physician-hospital management dialogue. *Surgery* 137:132-140.

Cohn KH. 2005. Embracing Complexity, from Cohn KH. *Better Communication for Better Care: Mastering Physician-Administrator Collaboration*, Chicago, Health Administration Press, Pp. 30-38.

Coile RC. 1994. Movement toward managed care leads to shifts in organizational cultures. *Georgia Hospitals Today* 38:4-6.

Coleman J, Katz E, Menzel. December 1957. "The diffusion of an innovation among physicians." *Sociometry* 20(4): 253-270.

Collins JC, Porras JI. 1997. Built to Last. HarperBusiness: New York.

Collins J. 2001. Good to Great. HarperBusiness, New York.

Command Paper: CM 5207. July 2001. The Inquiry into the management of care of children receiving complex heart surgery at the Bristol Royal Infirmary—Final Report. Accessed March 2006 at: www.bristol-inquiry.org.uk.

Conger JA, Kanungo RN. 1988. The empowerment process: Integrating theory and practice. *Academy of Management Review* 13: 471-482.

Conlin M. Smashing the Clock. YahooBusinessOnLine accessed December 8, 2006 at: http://biz.yahoo.com/special/allbiz120606_article1.html.

Connelly LM, Bott M, Hoffart N, Taunton RL. 1997. Methodologic triangulation in a study of nurse retention. *Nursing Research* Sept/Oct 46(5): 299-302.

Conner D. 1990. Corporate culture: Healthcare's change master. *Healthcare Executive* 5: 28-9.

Consumer Reports February 2007. Get better care from your doctor. Accessed January 4, 2006 at: www.ConsumerReports

Cooke R, Szumal J. 1991. Measuring normative beliefs and shared behavioral expectations in organizations: The Reliability and Validity of the Organizational Culture Inventory. *Psychological Reports* 72: 1299-1330.

Cooke RA, Szumal J. 2000. Using the organizational culture inventory to understand operating cultures of organizations. In Neal M. Ashkanasy, Celeste P. M. Wilderon, and Mark

F. Peterson (Eds.), Handbook of organizational culture and climate (pp. 147-162). Thousand Oaks, CA: Sage Publications.

Cotton JL, Vollrath DA, Froggatt KL, Lengnick-Hall ML, Jennings KR. 1988. Employee participation: Diverse forms and different outcomes. *Academy of Management Review*, 13(1): 8-22.

Coulson JD, Seddon MR, Readdy WF. March 2008. Advancing Safety in pediatric cardiology—Approaches Developed in Aviation. *Congenital Cardiology Today*, Vol 6, No. 3, Pp 1-10.

Coutu DL. 2002. The anxiety of Learning. [Interview with Edgar Schein]. *Harvard Business Review* March, pp 100-106.

Covey, SR 1989. The Seven Habits of Highly Effective People. Simon & Schuster: New York.

Cox, A. 1987. The Court and the Constitution. Houghton Miflin: Boston.

Cuny J (2005) Failure to Rescue—2004 Benchmarking Project. Accessed June 2005 at: www.uhc.edu.

D'Aunno T, Alexander JA, Laughlin C. 1996. Business as usual? Changes in Health Care's workforce and organization of work. *Hospital and Health Services Administration* 16: 3-18.

Dalton DR, Todor WD. 1979. Turnover turned over: An expanded and positive perspective. *Academy of Management Review* 4: 225-35.

Damasio AR. 1994. Descartes' Error: Emotion, Reason and the Human Brain. Avon Books: New York.

Danzon PM. 1985. Medical Malpractice: Theory, Evidence and Public Policy. Harvard University Press, Cambridge, MA.

Danzon PM. 1986. New evidence on the frequency and severity of medical malpractice claims. Rand Corporation, Santa Monica, CA. R-3410-ICJ.

Daschle, T Greenberger, SS, Lambrew JM. 2008. Critical: What We Can Do About the Health-Care Crisis. New York: St. Martin's Press.

Davidson M. 1983. Uncommon Sense—The Life and Thought of Ludwig von Bertalanffy (1901-1972), Father of General Systems Theory. Tarcher, Inc., Los Angeles.

Dauten D. 2001. The cost of being ordinary. Dale@dauten.com

Davies HTO, Nutley SM, Mannion R. 2000. Organizational Culture and Quality of Health Care. *Quality in Health Care* 9: 111-9.

Davis TRV: "Managing Culture at the Bottom" pages 163-182. In: Kilmann RH, Saxton MJ, Serpa R, et al (1985) Gaining Control of the Corporate Culture. San Francisco: Jossey-Bass.

Davis SM: "Culture Is Not Just and Internal Affair" pages 137-147. In: Kilmann RH, Saxton MJ, Serpa R, et al (1985) Gaining Control of the Corporate Culture. San Francisco: Jossey-Bass.

Deal TE, Kennedy AA. 1982. Corporate Culture: Rites and Rituals of Corporate Life. Perseus Publishing, Cambridge, MA.

Deal TE: "Cultural Change: Opportunity, Silent Killer, or Metamorphosis?" pages 292-331. In: Kilmann RH, Saxton MJ, Serpa R, et al (1985) Gaining Control of the Corporate Culture. San Francisco: Jossey-Bass.

Deal TE, Kennedy AA. 1999. The New Corporate Cultures. Perseus Books, Reading MA.

Deems RS. 1999. Calculating true cost of employee turnover. *Balance* 3(3): 13

Degeling P, Kennedy J, Hill, M. 1998. Do Professional Subcultures Set the Limits of Hospital Reform? *Clinician in Management* 7: 89-98.

Denison DR, Spreitzer GM. 1991. Organizational culture and organizational development: a competing values approach, *Research in Organizational Change and Development,* 5:1-21.

Desjardins RE. 1997. Does your corporate culture contribute to the problem? *Food & Drug Law Journal* 52:169-71.

Dilts DM, Sandler AB. 2006. The "Invisible" Barriers to Clinical Trials: The impact of Structural, Infrastructural, and Procedural Barriers to Opening Oncology Clinical Trials. *Journal Clinical Oncology*, 24(28): 4545-52.

Dixon K. 2004. HMOs bringing back unpopular cost controls-Survey. *Reuters*, 8/10/04. Accessed 8/10/04 at: http://news.yahoo.com/news? tmpl=story&cid=571&u= /nm/20040811/hl_nm/health_hmos_study.

Dobyns L. March 20, 2006. How hospitals heal themselves. Accessed 9/16/06 at: www.managementwisdom.com/goodnews.html.

Donabedian A. 1985. Explorations in Quality Monitoring and Assessment and Monitoring—Volume III, The Methods and Findings of Quality Assessment and Monitoring: An Illustrated Analysis. Health administration Press, Ann Arbor, MI.

Douglas CH, Higgins A, Dabbs, C, Walbank M. 2004. Health impact assessment for the sustainable futures of Salford. *Journal of Epidemiology and Community Health* 58: 642-648.

Dowd S, Davidhizar R. 1997. Change management—organizational culture as change factor. *Administrative Radiology Journal* 16:20-5.

Drake D, Fitzgerald S, Jaffe M. 1993. Hard Choices—Health Care at What Cost? Andrews & McMeel: Kansas City.

Droste TM. 1996. Merging corporate cultures in integrated systems. *Medical Network Strategy Report* 5:1-3.

Dwore, RB Dwore RB, Murray BP. 1989. Turnover at the top: Utah hospital CEOs in a turbulent era. *Hospital Health Services Administration* Fall, 34(3): 333-351.

Dyer, Jr. WG: The Cycle of Cultural Evolution in Organizations, pages 200-229. In: Kilmann RH, Saxton MJ, Serpa R, et al (1985) Gaining Control of the Corporate Culture. San Francisco: Jossey-Bass.

Dyer, WG. 1987. Team building: Issues and alternatives (2nd Edition). Reading, MA: Addison Wesley Publishing Company.

Ebon M. 1987. The Soviet Propaganda Machine. McGraw-Hill: New York.

Edmondson AC. 1996. Learning from mistakes is easier said than done: Group and organizational influences on the detection and correction of human error. *Journal of Applied Behavioral Science,* 32(1): 5-28.

Edmondson, AC. 2008. The Competitive Imperative of Learning. *Harvard Business Review* July-August: 60-67.

Edmonton TV. Opposition demand health care review. Accessed 3/11/11: http://calgary.ctv.ca/servlet/an/local/ CTVNews/20110311/CGY_health_care_110311/2011031 1/?hub=CalgaryHome.

Ellis, Libby et al. November 30, 2017. Trends in Cancer Survival by Health Insurance Status in California from 1997 to 2014. *JAMA Oncology.*

Ellis SG, Weintraub W, Holmes D, Shaw R, Block PC, King SB. 1997. Relation of Operator Volume and Experience to Procedural Outcome of Percutaneous Coronary Revascularization at Hospitals with High Interventional Volumes. *Circulation* 95: 2479–84.

Engstrom P. 1995. Cultural differences can fray the knot after MDs, hospitals exchange vows. *Medical Network Strategy Report,* 4:1-5.

Epstein RA. 1999. Mortal Peril—Our Inalienable Right to Health Care? Perseus Books: Cambridge, MA.

Eubanks P. 1991. Identifying your hospital's corporate culture. *Hospitals* 65: 46.

European Observatory on Health Care Systems 2000. Health Care Systems in Transition: Belgium. Copenhagen: World Health Organization. Accessed on February 10, 2006 at: http://www.euro.who.int/document/e71203.pdf.

Evans M. October 18, 2004. For a limited time only. *Modern Healthcare.* 34 (42): 6-8.

Executive Order 13765. 2017. "Minimizing the Economic Burden of the Patient Protection and Affordable Care Act Pending Repeal." *The White House.*

Executive Order 13828. 2018. "Reducing Poverty in America by Promoting Opportunity and Economic mobility." *The White House.*

Fallin, Mary. March 5, 2018. "Executive Order 2018-05."

Feldstein PJ. 2005. *Health Care Economics*, 6th ed. Thomson Delmar Learning. Clifton, NY. Pp. 207-208.

Fennell ML, Alexander J. September 1987. Organization boundary spanning and institutionalized environments. *Academy of Management Journal* 30: 456-476.

Ferlie E, Fitzgerald L, Wood M. 2000. Getting evidence into clinical practice: an organizational behavior perspective. *Journal of Health Services Research & Policy* 5(2): 96-102.

Ferlie EB, Shortell SM. 2001. Improving the quality of health care in the United Kingdom and the United States: A framework for change. *Millbank Quarterly* 79(2): 281-315.

Ferrara-Love R. 1997. Changing organizational culture to implement organizational change. *Journal of Perianesthesia Nursing* 12: 12-6.

Fickeisen DH. Winter 1991. Learning How to Learn, An Interview with Kathy Greenberg. The Learning Revolution (IC#27) by the Context Institute. Page 42. www.context.org/ICLIB/IC27/Greenbrg.htm. Accessed December 2004.

Finley, Allysia. July 25, 2018. ObamaCare Is Robbing Medicaid's Sickest Patients. *Wall Street Journal.*

Fiol CM, O'Connor EJ, Aguinis. 2001. All for one and one for all? The development and transfer of power across organizational levels. *Academy of Management Review*, 26(2): 224-242.

Fitzgerald FS. 1936. The Crack-Up. New Directions Books: New York. Reprinted 1945.

Flowers VS, Hughes CL. July/August 1973. Why employees stay. *Harvard Business Review* pp. 49-60.

Fletcher B, Jones F. 1992. Measuring Organizational Culture: The Cultural Audit. *Managerial Auditing Journal* 7 (6): 30-6.

Forrester JW. 1971. The counterintuitive behavior of social systems. *Technology Review,* 73(3): 52-68.

Franczyk A. 2000. Turnover in hospital CEOs brings change to healthcare industry. *Business First.* Buffalo: Jul24, 2000. Vol 12, Iss. 44, pp1-2.

Freiberg K, Freiberg J. 1996. Nuts! Southwest Airlines' Crazy Recipe for Business and Personal Success. Broadway Books: New York.

Friedman EA, Adashi EY. December 15, 2010. The right to health as the unheralded narrative of health care reform. *Journal of the American Medical Association* 304(23): 2639-2640.

Galloro V. February 19, 2001. Staffing outlook grim-High turnover expected to continue in skilled nursing, assisted living. *Modern Healthcare* 31(8): 64.

Garside P. 1998. Organizational context for quality: Lesson from the fields of organizational development and change management. *Quality in Health Care* 7(Suppl): S8-15.

Garson A. 2001. The Edgar Mannheim Lecture: From white teeth to heart transplants: evolution in international concepts of the quality of healthcare. *Cardiology in the Young* 11: 601-608.

Gawande A. 12/30/07. A Lifesaving checklist. *NewYorkTimes. com* at: http://www.nytimes.com/2007/12/30/opinion/30gawande.html?_r=2&oref=slogin.

Gawande A. January 24, 2011. Can we lower medical costs by giving the neediest patients better care? *New Yorker Online*. Accessed March 7, 2011 at: http://www.newyorker.com/reporting/2011/01/24/110124fa_fact_gawande?currentPage=all.

Gawande A. May 26, 2011. Cowboys and Pit Crews. *The New Yorker*. Accessed at: http://www.newyorker.com/online/blogs/newsdesk/2011/05/atul-gawande-harvard-medical-school-commencement-address.html.

Gentry WD, Parkes KR. 1982. Psychologic stress in the ICU and non-intensive unit nursing: A review of the past decade. *Heart & Lung* 11(1): 43-47.

George JM, Jones GR. 1996. The experience and work and turnover intentions: Interactive effects of value attainment, job satisfaction, and positive mood. *Journal of Applied Psychology* 81(3): 318-325.

Gerowitz M, Lemieux-Charles L, Heginbothan C, and Johnson B. 1996. Top Management Culture and Performance in Canadian, UK and US Hospitals. *Health Services Management Research* 6 (3): 69-78.

Gibson, M., et al. 2018. "Welfare-to-work interventions and their effects on the mental and physical health of lone parents and their children." *Cochrane Database of Systematic Reviews* 2018(2).

Ginn, Vance, Waldman, Deane. August 12, 2017. The Senate's healthcare double whammy: fewer jobs and less care. *The Hill*.

Glaser S, Zamanou S, Hacker K. 1987. Measuring and Interpreting Organizational Culture. *Management communication quarterly* 1 (2): 173-98.

Glazner L. 1992. Understanding corporate cultures: use of systems theory and situational analysis. *American Association of Occupational Health Nurses Journal* 40:383-7.

Goldman RL. 1992. The reliability of peer assessment of quality of care. *Journal of the American Medical Association* 267(7): 958-960.

Goldman DP, McGlynn EA. 2005. US Health Care: Facts about Cost, Access and Quality. Rand Report CP484.1. Accessed December 29, 2006 at: www.rand.org/pubs/corporate-pubs/CP484.1.

Goldratt E, Cox J (1984). The Goal-A Process of Ongoing Improvement. North River Press, Great Barrington, MA.

Goldsmith J. 2003. Digital Medicine: Implications for Healthcare Leaders. Chicago: Health Administration Press.

Goldworth A. 2008. "Human rights and the right to health care." In: Weisstub DN, Diaz Pintos G. 2008. Autonomy and Human Rights in Health Care. Springer: The Netherlands.

Goodman EA, Boss RW. 1999. Burnout dimensions and voluntary and involuntary turnover in a health care setting. *Journal of Health & Human Services Administration* Spring, 21(4): 462-471.

Goodman J. November 8, 2010. Being stupid about prices. Accessed May 2011 at: http://healthblog.ncpa.org/stupid-about-prices.

Goodman JM, Jones GR. 1996. The experience and work and turnover intentions: Interactive effects of value attainment, job satisfaction, and positive mood. *Journal of Applied Psychology* 81(3): 318-325.

Goold M, Campbell A. 2002. Do you have a well-designed organization? *Harvard Business Review* March 117-124.

Gordon GG: "The Relationship of Corporate Culture to Industry Sector and Corporate Performance" pages 103-125. In: Kilmann RH, Saxton MJ, Serpa R, et al (1985) Gaining Control of the Corporate Culture. San Francisco: Jossey-Bass.

Gray AM, Phillips VL, Normand C. 1996. The costs of nursing turnover: Evidence from the British National Health Service. *Health Policy* 38: 117-128

Greco PJ, Eisenberg JM. 1993. Changing Physicians' Practices. *New England Journal of Medicine* 329(17): 1271-1274.

Greene J. February 6, 1995. Clinical integration increases profitability, efficiency—study. *Modern Healthcare*, page 39

Griffeth RW, Hom PW, Hall TE. 1981. How to estimate employee turnover costs. Personnel 58(4): 43-52.

Griffeth RW, Hom PW. 2001. Retaining Valued Employees. Sage Publications, Thousand Oaks, CA.

Groupman J. 2007. How Doctors Think. Houghton Miflin: New York.

Grout JR. 2003. Preventing medical errors by designing benign failures. *Joint Commission Journal on Quality and Safety* 29(7): 354-362.

Gustafson BM. 2001. Improving staff satisfaction ensures PFS success. *Healthcare Financial Management* 55(7): 66-68.

Hadley J, Mitchell JM, Sulmasy DP, Bloch MG. 1999. Perceived financial incentives, HMO market penetration, and physicians' practice styles and satisfaction. *Health Services Research* Vol. 34, #1, Part II: 307-321.

Haft H. The right to Basic Health Care is Afforded to Every Citizen of the United States. *Physician Executive* Jan-Feb 2003. http://findarticles.com/p/articles/mi_m0843/is_1_29/ai_96500897.

Haislmaier, Edmund. 2015. "2014 [Enrollment] Increase Due Almost Entirely to Medicaid Expansion." *Heritage Foundation*.

Hale C. May 7, 2003. NHS Chiefs 'forced into trickery.' *London Times*, P 6.

Hall ET, Hall MR. 1990. Understanding Cultural Differences. Intercultural Press, Yarmouth, Maine.

Hammer M, Champy J. 1994. Reengineering the Corporation-A Manifesto for Business Revolution. HarperBusiness, New York, NY.

Hammer M. 2001. The Agenda. Crown Business, New York.

Hannan, EL, Racz M, Kavey R-E, et al. 1998. Pediatric Cardiac Surgery: The Effect of Hospital and Surgeon Volume on In-hospital Mortality. *Pediatrics* 101(6): 963-69.

Hariri S, Prestipino AL, Rubash HE. April 2007. The Hospital-Physician Relationship: Past, Present and Future. *Clinical Orthopaedics and Related Research* 457: 78-86.

Harrison, R. 1972. Understanding Your Organization's Character. *Harvard Business Review* 5 (3): 119-28.

Hart, Angela. 2018. "More undocumented immigrants would qualify for health care in $250 million California plan." *Sacramento Bee.*

Hart LG, Robertson DG, Lishner DM, Rosenblatt RA. 1993. CEO turnover in rural northwest hospitals. *Hospital Health Services Administration* Fall; 38(3): 353-374.

Haskins, Ron. Testimony before House of Representatives Ways and Means Committee, on Effects of the 1996 Welfare Reform Law, July 19, 2006.

Haskins, Ron. Testimony before House of Representatives Ways and Means Committee, on Challenging Facing Low-income Individuals and Families, February 11, 2015.

Hatch AP. 2005. CBS abandons Murrow Ideals. *Albuquerque Journal* October 20; Page A13.

Hawkes, Nigel. January 18, 2002. Patients get power to select surgeons. *London Times*

Hayes, Tara O'Neill. 2017. "How Many Are Newly Insured as a Result of the ACA?" *American Action Forum.*

Heinlein R. 1963. Glory Road. Avon Books: New York. Page 253.

Heinlein, R.1966. The Moon Is A Harsh Mistress. Berkley Publishing Corp: New York.

Henninger D. January 10, 2003. Marcus Welby doesn't live here anymore. *Wall Street Journal*, Page A10.

Herzberg F. 1968. One more time: How do you motivate employees? *Harvard Business Review* Reprint RO301F in *Best of HBR* January 2003 pp. 3-11.

Herzlinger RE. 1997. Market-Driven Health Care. Addison-Wesley Publ., Reading MA.

Herzlinger RE. November 26, 2003. Back in the USS.R. *Wall Street Journal*, Opinion, Vol 240, A16.

Heskett JL, Sasser WE, Schlesinger LA: The Service Profit Chain, Free Press, NY, 1997.

HHS REPORT: "Average Health Insurance Premiums Doubled Since 2013," May 2017.

Hill LD, Madara JL. November 2, 2005. Role of the Urban Academic Medical Center in US Health Care. *JAMA* 294(17): 2219-2220.

Hilts PJ. June 23, 1993. Health-care Chiefs' pay rises at issue." *New York Times*, pg D2.

Hint. 2017. "Direct Primary Care Trends Report 2017.

Hoban CJ. 2002. From the lab to the clinic: Integration of pharmacogenics into clinical development. *Pharmacogenics* 3(4): 429-436.

Hock D. 1999. Birth of the Chaordic Age. Berrett-Koehler: San Francisco, CA.

Hofstede G, Neuijen B, Ohayv DD, Sanders G. 1990. Measuring organizational cultures: A qualitative and quantitative study across twenty cases. *Administrative Science Quarterly* 35:286-316.

Horton, Nicholas. 2015. Shocking report reveals rampant welfare fraud in Arkansas. *Townhall.com*.

Horton, Nicholas. November 23, 2016. "Hundreds on Medicaid waiting list in Illinois die while waiting for care." *IllinoisPolicy. com*.

Howard PK. July 31, 2002. There is no 'right to sue.' *Wall Street Journal*, Page 13.

Hughes L. 1990. Assessing organizational culture: Strategies for external consultant. *Nursing Forum* 25 (1): 15-19.

Hume SK. 1990. Strengthening the corporate culture. *Health Progress* 71:15-6, 19.

Huselid MA, Jackson SE, Schuler RS. 1997. Technical and strategic human resource management effectiveness as determinants of firm performance. *Academy of Management Journal* 40(1): 171-188.

Hutchinson J, Runge W, Mulvey M, et al. 2004. *Burkholderia cepacia* infections associated with intrinsically contaminated ultrasound gel: The role of microbial degradation of parabens. *Infection Control and Hospital Epidemiology* 25: 291-296

Iglehart J. 1998. Forum on the future of academic medicine: Session III—Getting from Here to There. *Academic Medicine* 73 (2): 146-151

Ingersoll GL, Kirsch JC, Merk SE, et al. 2000. Relationship of Organizational culture and Readiness for Change to Employee Commitment to the Organization. *Journal of Nursing Admin* 30 (1); 11-20.

Ingram, Jonathan. 2015. "Stop the scam — How to prevent welfare fraud in your state." Foundation for Government Accountability.

Irvine DM, Evans MG. 1995. Job satisfaction and Turnover among nurses: Integrating research findings across studies. *Nursing Research* July/August 44(4): 246-253.

Jacobs DC. 2004. A pragmatist approach to integrity in business ethics. *Journal of Management Inquiry* September 13(3): 215-223.

Jain KK. 2005. Personalised medicine for cancer: from drug development into clinical practice. *Expert Opinions in Pharmacotherapy* 6(9): 1463-1476.

Janssen PPM, de Jonge J, Bakker AB. 1999. Specific determinants of intrinsic work motivation, burnout and turnover intentions: a study among nurses. *Journal of Advanced Nursing* 29(6): 1360-1369.

Jenkins KJ, Gauvreau K, Newburger JW, et al. 2002. Consensus-based method for risk adjustment for surgery for congenital heart disease. *Journal of Thoracic & Cardiovascular Surgery* January 123: 110-118.

Jha AK, Perlin JB, Kizer KW, Dudley RA. May 29, 2003. Effect of the transformation of the Veterans Affairs Health Care System and the quality of care. *New England Journal of Medicine* 348(2): 2218-2227.

Jiang HJ, Friedman B, Begun JW. 2006. Factors Associated with High-Quality/Low-Cost Hospital Performance. *Journal of Health Care Finance* Spring: 39-51.

Johnson DE. 1997. Medical group cultures pose big challenges. *Health Care Strategic Management* 15:2-3.

Johnson J, Billingsley M. 1997. Reengineering the corporate culture of hospitals." *Nursing & Health Care Perspectives* 18:316-21.

Johnson L. 1999. Cutting costs by managing turnover. *Balance, The Journal of the American College of Health Care Administrators*. Sept/Oct 1999 pp 21-23.

Johnson, Rep. Nancy. February 2001. Congressional Outlook: Nursing Shortages. *Hospital Outlook* 4(2): 7.

Johnson S. 2001. Emergence. New York: Simon & Schuster, 2001.

Joiner KA, Wormsley S. March 2005. Strategies for Defining Financial Benchmarks for the Research Mission in Academic Health Centers. *Academic Medicine* 80(3): 211-217.

Joiner KA. March 2005. A Strategy for allocating central funds to support new faculty recruitment. *Academic Medicine* 80(3): 218-224.

Joiner KA. July 2004. Sponsored-Research Funding by Newly Recruited Assistant Professors: Can It Be Modeled as a Sequential Series of Uncertain Events? *Academic Medicine* 79(7): 633-643.

Joiner KA. July 2004. Using Utility Theory to Optimize a Salary Incentive Plan for Grant-Funded Faculty, *Academic Medicine* 79(7): 652-660.

Jollis JG, Peterson ED, DeLong ER, et al. 1994. The Relation Between the Volume of Coronary Angioplasty Procedures at Hospitals Treating Medicare Beneficiaries and Short-Term Mortality. *New England Journal of Medicine* 331: 1625-29.

Jones WT. 1961. The Romantic Syndrome: Toward a new method in cultural anthropology and the history of ideas. The Hague: Martinus Wijhaff.

Jones CB. 1990a. Staff nurse turnover costs: Part I, a conceptual model. *Journal of Nursing Administration,* 20(4): 18-22. AND

Jones CB. 1990b. Staff nurse turnover costs: Part II, measurement and results. *Journal of Nursing Administration,* 20(5): 27-32.

Jones CB. 1992. Calculating and Updating Nursing Turnover Costs." *Nursing Economic$* January/February 10(1): 39-45, 78.

Jones KR, DeBaca V, Yarbrough M. 1997. Organizational culture assessment before and after implementing patient-focused care. *Nursing Economics* 1997; 15:73-80.

Jones WJ. 2000. The 'Business'—or 'Public Service'—of Healthcare. *Journal of Healthcare Management,* 45(5): 290-293.

Jorgensen A: Creating changes in the corporate culture: case study. *American Association of Occupational Health Nurses Journal* 1991; 39:319-21.

Jung CG. 1973. Four archetypes: Mother/Rebirth/Spirit/ Trickster. Princeton University Press: Princeton, NJ.

Jurkiewicz CL, Knouse SB, Giacalone RA (March/April 2001) "When an employee leaves: The effectiveness of clinician exit interviews and surveys." *Clinical Leadership Management Review* 15(2): 81-84.

Kaiser Family Foundation, March 2009. Health Care Costs—A Primer. Accessed March 2009 at: www.kff.org.

Kan JS, White RI, Mitchell SE, Gardner TJ. 1982. Percutaneous balloon valvuloplasty: a new method for treating congenital pulmonary valve stenosis. *New England Journal of Medicine* 307: 540-542.

Kallestad B. Fall 2006. *Leadership Quarterly*, Associated Press Report accessed January 1, 2007 at: http://news.yahoo.com/s/ap/bad_bosses

Karcz A, Korn R, Burke MC, et al. (1996) Malpractice Claims Against Emergency Physicians in Massachusetts: 1975-1993. *American Journal of Emergency Medicine* 14: 341-345.

Kauffman, Draper. 1980. Systems One: An Introduction to Systems Thinking. SA Carlton, Minneapolis, MN.

Kauffman SA. 1995. At Home in the Universe. Oxford University Press, NY.

Keeler EB, Brook RH, Goldberg GA, Kamberg CJ, Newhouse JP (1985) "How free care reduced hypertension in the Health Insurance Experiment." *Journal of the American Medical Association* Oct. 11, 1985; Vol. 254: 1926-1931.

Keeton WP, Dobbs DB, Keeton RE, Owen DG. 1984. *Prosser and Keeton on The Law of Torts*. Fifth Edition. West Publishing Co., St. Paul, MN.

Kellerman B. 2007. What every leader needs to know about followers. *Harvard Business Review* December, pp. 84-91.

Kerr S. 1975. On the folly of rewarding A While hoping for B. *Academy of Management Journal* 18: 769-783.

Kesner KA, Calkin JD. 1986. Critical care nurses' intent to stay in their positions. *Research in Nursing & Health* 9: 3-10.

Kessler DP, McClellan MB. 2002. How liability law affects medical productivity. *Journal of Medical Economics* 21(6): 931-955.

Kiel JM. 1998. Using data to reduce employee turnover. *Health Care Supervisor* 16(4): 12-19.

Kilmann RH, Saxton MJ, Serpa R, et al. 1985. Gaining Control of the Corporate Culture. San Francisco: Jossey-Bass. See: Kilmann RH: "Five Steps of Closing Culture Gaps" pages 351-369 and Kilmann RH, Saxton MJ and Serpa R: "Conclusion: Why Culture Is Not Just a Fad," pages 421-432.

Kinard J, Little B. 1999. Are hospitals facing a critical shortage of skilled workers? *Health Care Supervisor* 17(4): 54-62.

King L. 1963. The Growth of Medical Thought. University of Chicago Press: Chicago.

Kissick WL. 1995. Medicine and Management – Bridging the cultural gaps. *Physician Executive* 21:3-6.

Kite M. June 03, 2003. Fat people will have to diet if they want to see the doctor. *London Times*.

Klaasen P. March 14, 2007. Accessed at: www.cnn.com/2007/HEALTH/04/04/uninsured.dead.ap/index.htm.

Klein LW, Schaer GL, Calvin JE, et al. 1997. Does Low Individual Operator Coronary Interventional Procedural Volume Correlate with Worse Institutional Procedural Outcome? *Journal of the American College of Cardiology* 30, no. 4: 870-77.

Klienke JD. 1998. Bleeding Edge-The Business of Health Care in the New Century. Aspen Publishers, Gaithersburg, MD.

Klienke JD. September/October 2005. Dot-Gov: Market failure and the creation of a national health information technology system. *Health Affairs* 24(5): 1246-1262.

Klingle RS, Burgoon M, Afifi W, Callister M. 1995. Rethinking how to measure organizational culture in the hospital setting. The Hospital Culture Scale. *Evaluation & the Health Professions* 18:166-86.

Kosmoski KA, Calkin JD. 1986. Critical care nurses' intent to stay in their positions. *Research in Nursing & Health* 9: 3-10.

Kotter JP, Schlesinger LA. 1979. Choosing strategies for change." *Harvard Business Review* Mar-Apr 57(2): 106-114

Kotter JP, Heskett JL. 1992. Corporate Culture and Performance. Free Press: New York.

Kouzes JM, Posner BZ. 1997. The Leadership Challenge; Jossey-Bass Inc., San Francisco

Krackhardt D, Porter LW. 1985. When friends leave: A structural analysis of the relationship between turnover and stayers' attitudes. *Administrative Science Quarterly*, 30, 42-61.

Kraman SS, Hamm G. 1999. Risk management: Extreme honesty may be the best policy. *Annals of Internal Medicine* 131(12): 963-967.

Kravitz RL, Rolph JE, Petersen L. 1997. Omission-Related Malpractice Claims and the Limits of Defensive Medicine. *Medical Care Res & Review* 54: 456-471.

Krauthammer C. 1998. Driving the best doctors away. *Washington Post* January 9; p A21.

Kübler-Ross, E. 1969. On Death and Dying. Touchstone: New York.

Lacour-Gayet F, Clarke D, Jacobs J, et al. 2004. The Aristotle Score: a complexity-adjusted method to evaluate surgical results. *European Journal of Cardio-Thoracic Surgery* 25: 911-924.

Landis SE. January 3, 2006. Do the Poor deserve life support? Accessed December12, 2006 at www.slate.com/toolbar.aspx?action.

Landon BE, Reschovsky J, Blumenthal D. 2003. Changes in career satisfaction among primary care and specialist physicians, 1997-2001. *JAMA* 289(4): 442-449.

Landro, Laura. December 22, 2003. Six prescriptions for what's ailing US Health care. *Wall Street Journal* Vol 242 #122, pp. A1 & A10.

Langer E. 1997. The Power of Mindful Learning. Perseus Books: New York.

LaPar, Damien, et al. September 2010. Primary Payer Status Affects Mortality for Major Surgical Operations. *Annals of Surgery* 252(3): 544-551.

Langwell KM, Werner JL. 1984. Regional Variations in the Determinants of Professional Liability Claims. *Journal of Health Politics, Policy and Law* 9:475-88.

Laurance J. December 6, 2004. NHS Revolution: nurses to train as surgeons. *The Independent* (London)

Lawry TC. May 1995. Making culture a forethought. *Health Progress* 76(4): 22-25, 48

Lazlo E. 1972. The Systems View of the World. G Braziller: New York.

Leape LL. December 21, 1994. Error in Medicine. *JAMA* 272(3): 1851-1857.

Lee RT, Ashforth BE. 1996. A meta-analytic examination of the correlates of the three dimensions of job burnout. *Journal of Applied Psychology* 81: 123-133.

Lerner J. 1997. *The Rush Initiative for Mediation of Medical Malpractice Claims.* 11 CBA Record 40.

Levering R, Moskovitz M. 1993. *The 100 Best Companies to Work for in America*; Doubleday, New York.

Levinson W, Roter DL, Mullooly JP, et al. 1997. Physician-Patient Communication: The Relationship with Malpractice Claims Among Primary Care Physicians and Surgeons. *Journal of the American Medical Association* 277: 553-559.

Levitt S, Dubner S. 2005. Freakonomics—A Rogue Economist Explores the Hidden Side of Everything. Harper Collins: New York.

Lewin K. 1947. Frontiers in group dynamics. *Human Relations*, Volume 1, pp. 5-41.

Linn A. February 12, 2005. Biggest Airbus Jet is Too Big. *Albuquerque Journal*, No. 43, C-1. 4

Lisney B, Allen C. 1993. Taking a snapshot of cultural change. *Personnel Management* 25 (2): 38-41.

Litwinenko A, Cooper CL: "The impact of trust status on corporate culture." *Journal of Management in Medicine* 1994; 8:8-17.

Localio AR, Lawthers AG, Brennan TA, et al. 1991. Relation between malpractice claims and adverse events due to negligence: Results of the Harvard Medical Practice Study III. *New England Journal of Medicine,* 325: 245-251.

Loop FD. 2001. On medical management. *Journal of Thoracic and Cardiovascular Surgery,* 121(4): S25-S28.

Lopez-Bauman, Naomi, Rea Hederman, Lindsay Boyd Killen. 2017. "Medicaid Waiver Toolkit." State Policy Network Healthcare Working Group.

Lorsch JW: "Strategic Myopia: Culture as an Invisible Barrier to Change" pages 84-102. In: Kilmann RH, Saxton MJ, Serpa R, et al (1985) Gaining Control of the Corporate Culture. San Francisco: Jossey-Bass.

Louis MR: "Sourcing Workplace Cultures: Why, When, and How" pages 126-136-102. In: Kilmann RH, Saxton MJ, Serpa R, et al (1985) Gaining Control of the Corporate Culture. San Francisco: Jossey-Bass.

Luft HS, Bunker, Enthoven AC. 1979. Should operations be regionalized? The empirical relation between surgical volume and mortality. *New England Journal of Medicine,* Dec 20; 301(25): 1364-69.

Luft, HS. 2003. From observing the relationship between volume and outcome to making policy recommendations— Comments on Sheikh. *Medical Care* 41(10): 1118-1122.

Lurie N, Manning WG, Peterson C, Goldberg GA, Phelps CA, Lilliard L. 1987. Preventive Care: Do we practice what we preach? *American Journal of Public Health* 77:801-804.

Maarse H, Paulus A. Has solidarity survived? A comparative analysis of the effect of social health insurance reform in four European countries. *Journal of Health, Politics, Policy and Law* 2003; 28(4): 585-614.

Machiavelli N. 1513. The Prince. Wordsworth Editions, Hertfordshire, England, 1993.

Mackenzie S. 1995. Surveying the organizational culture in a NHS trust. *Journal of Medical Management* 9(6): 69-77.

Mackey J. August 11, 2009. The Whole Foods Alternative to Obamacare. *Wall Street Journal.* Online. http://online.wsj.com/article/SB10001424052970204251404574342170072865070.html.

Maclean, N. 1992. Young Men and Fire. University of Chicago: Chicago. Mahony L, Sleeper LA, Anderson PAW, et al. 2006. Pediatric Heart Network: A primer for the conduct of multicenter studies in children with congenital & acquired heart disease. *Pediatric Cardiology* 27: 191-198.

Malcolm L, Wright L, Barnett, Hendry C. 2003. Building a successful partnership between management and clinical leadership: experience from New Zealand. *British Medical Journal* 326: 653-654. Downloaded 31 August 2006 from doi:10.1136/bmj.326.7390.653.

Manger LN 2005. A History of Medicine. Taylor & Francis: New York.

Mann EE, Jefferson KJ. Retaining staff: Using turnover indices and surveys. *Journal of Nursing Administration* 1988; 18(7,8): 17-23.

Mano-Negrin R. 2001. An occupational preference model of turnover behavior: The case of Israel's medical sector employees. *Journal of Management in Medicine* 15(2): 106-114.

Marmot M. 2004. The Status Syndrome—How Social Standing Affects Our Health and Longevity. Holt & Co.: New York.

Marsh R Mannari H. 1977. Organizational commitment and turnover: A predictive study. *Administrative Science Quarterly* 22: 57-75.

Martin, N. June 4, 2007. "Smokers who won't quit denied surgery" by Nicole Martin in the *Daily Telegraph Today*, June 4, 2007, at: http://www.telegraph.co.uk/global/ main.jhtml?xml=/ global/2007/06/04/nhealth04.xml.

Martin TE. 1979. A contextual model of employee turnover intentions. *Academy of Management Journal* 22(2): 313-324.

Martin HJ: "Managing Specialized Corporate Cultures," pages 148-162. In: Kilmann RH, Saxton MJ, Serpa R, et al (1985) Gaining Control of the Corporate Culture. San Francisco: Jossey-Bass.

Maslow AH. 1943. A theory of human motivation. *Psychological Review* 50: 370-396.

Matthews, M. June 2, 2011. Irrational exuberance and accountable care organizations. Accessed 6/3/11 at: http://blogs.forbes. com/merrill matthews/2011/06/02/irrational-exuberance-and-accountable-care-organizations.

Matus JC, Frazer GH. 1996. Job satisfaction among selected hospital CEOs." *The Health Care Supervisor* September 15(1): 41-60.

May L. 1993. Institutions and the transformation of personal values. Are the traditional values of caring and service in jeopardy? *Clinical Laboratory Management Review* 7:191-3.

Matus JC, Frazer GH. 1996. Job satisfaction among selected hospital CEOs. *The Health Care Supervisor* September 15(1): 41-60.

McCallum KL. May 7, 2001. All the good doctors always leave. *Medical Economics* 78(9): 55-6, 58, 61.

McConnell CR. 1999. Staff turnover: Occasional friend, frequent foe, and continuing frustration. *Health Care Manager* 18(1): 1-13.

McDaniel RR. 1997. Strategic Leadership: A View from quantum and chaos theories. *Health Care Management Review* 22(1) 21-37.

McDaniel RR, Driebe DJ. 2001. Complexity Science and Health Care Management. *Advances in Health Care Management* 2: 11-36.

McFadden KL, Towell ER, Stock GN. 2004. Critical success factors for controlling and managing Hospital Errors. *Quality Management Journal* 2004; 11(1) 61-73.

McGinn R. May 10, 2006. Malpractice Caps Limit Care. *Albuquerque Journal*, #130, Page A11.

McGrath PD, Wennberg DE, Malenka DJ, et al. 1998. Operator Volume and Outcome in 12,998 Percutaneous Coronary Interventions. *Journal of American College of Cardiology* 31(3): 570–76.

McIntyre N, Popper KB. 1989. The critical attitude in medicine: the need for a new ethics. *British Medical Journal* 287:1919-1923.

McMurray, AJ. 2003. The relationship between organizational climate and organizational culture. *Journal of the American Academy of Business*, 3: 1-8.

McSwane, J. David, Chavez, Andrew. June 3,4,5,6,7, 2018. A Preventable Tragedy; Skimping on Care; Texas pays billions for 'sham' networks; Gloss-over of the Horror; and Parents vs. the Austin machine (Part 5 of 5). *Dallas Morning News*.

"Medicaid at 50. 2015." Kaiser Commission on Medicaid and the Uninsured. Accessed August 2018 at: http://files.kff.org/attachment/report-medicaid-at-50

Medicaid Law - Hospital Insurance Program. 1965. Public Law 89-97.

Melcher AJ (1976) Participation: A critical review of research findings. *Human Resource Management*. Summer: 12-21.

Melville A. 1980. Job satisfaction in general practice: Implications for prescribing. *Social Sciences & Medicine* 14A (6): 495-499.

Merritt Hawkins. 2015. "Physician Access Index–A State-by-State Compilation of Benchmarks and Metrics Influencing Patient Access to Physicians and Advanced Practitioners

Merritt Hawkins. 2017. Survey of Physician Appointment Wait Times, 2017.

Merry M. 1998. Will you manage your organization's culture, or will it manage you? *Integrated Healthcare Report* pp. 1-11.

Merry MD. 2004. What Deming Says. One of four essays on Can the gurus' concepts cure healthcare? *Quality Progress* September pp. 28-30.

Meschievitz CS. 1994. Efficacious or Precarious? Comments on the Processing and Resolution of Medical Malpractice Claims in the United States, 3 *Annals of Health Law* 123, 127-130.

Messinger DS, Bauer CR, Das A, et al. 2004. The maternal lifestyle study: Cognitive, motor, and behavioral outcomes of cocaine-exposed and opiate-exposed infants through three years of age. *Pediatrics* 113: 1677-168.

Metzloff TB. 1992. *Alternate Dispute Resolution Strategies in Medical Malpractice.* 9 Alaska L. Rev. 429, 431.

Metzloff TB. 1996. *The Unrealized Potential of Malpractice Arbitration,* 31 Wake Forest L. Rev. 203, 204, 1996.

Metzloff TB. 1997. *Empirical Perspectives on Mediation and Malpractice.* 60-WTR Law & Contemp. Probs. 107, 110-113. *See also,* N.C. Gen. Stat. § 7A-38.1 (1998).

Meyer, Bruce D., and James X. Sullivan. 2005. *The Well-Being of Single-Mother Families After Welfare Reform.* The Brookings Institution.

Millenson ML. 1999. Demanding Medical Excellence: Doctors and accountability in the Information Age. University of Chicago Press.

Millenson, ML. 2003. The Silence. *Health Affairs* 22(2): 103-112.

Miller, J 1995. Lockheed Martin's Skunk Works. Midland Publishers: Leicester, England.

Miller RH, Lipton HL, Duke KS, Luft HS. 1996. Update Special Report, The San Diego Health Care System: A Snapshot of Change. *Health Affairs* 15.1: 224-229.

Miller MM. December 25, 2003. Don't look for responsible leadership under tree. *Albuquerque Journal* Vol 358, A12.

Miller WL, Crabtree BF, McDaniel R, et al. May 1998. Understanding change in primary care practice using complexity theory. *Journal of Family Practice* 46(5): 369-376.

Mingardi A. November 17, 2006. A drug price path to avoid. *Albuquerque Journal*, A13.

Mintzberg H. 1983. Structuring of Organizations. Englewood Cliff: Prentice Hall.

Mirvis PH Lawler EE. 1977. Measuring the financial impact of employee attitudes. *Journal of Applied Psychology* 62:1-18.

Mitroff II and Kilmann RH: "Corporate Taboos and the Key to Unlocking Culture," pages 184-199. In: Kilmann RH, Saxton MJ, Serpa R, et al (1985) Gaining Control of the Corporate Culture. San Francisco: Jossey-Bass.

Mobley WH, Horner SO, Hollingsworth AT. 1978. Evaluation of precursors of hospital employee turnover. *Journal of Applied Psychology* 63(4): 408-414.

Mobley WH. 1982. Employee Turnover: Causes, Consequences and Control. Addison-Wesley, Reading, MA.

Moffit RE. Dec 23, 2010. Doctors, Patients, and the New Medicare Provisions. Heritage Foundation lectures #1174 (September 23, 2010): 1-8. Accessed January 2011 at: http://report.heritage.org/h1174.

Moore WW. 1991. Corporate culture: modern day rites & rituals." *Healthcare Trends & Transition* 2:8-10, 12-3, 32-3.

Morrissey, E. November 15, 2012. What free market medicine looks like. Accessed December 2012 at: http://hotair.com/archives/2012/11/15/video-what-free-market-medicine-looks-like.

Mosca L, Appel LJ, Benjamin EJ et al. 2004. Evidence-based guidelines for cardiovascular disease prevention in women. American Heart Association scientific statement. *Arteriosclerosis Thrombosis and Vascular Biology* Mar; 24(3): 29-50.

Mott DA. 2000. Pharmacist job turnover, length of service, and reasons for leaving, 1983-1997. *Amer Journal of Health-System Pharmacy* 57(10): 975-984.

Mowday RT, Steers RM, Porter LW. 1979. The measurement of organizational commitment. *Journal of Vocational Behavior* 14: 224-27.

Mowday RT. 1981. Viewing turnover from the perspective of those who remain: The relationship of job attitudes to attributions of the causes of turnover. *Journal of Applied Psychology* 66(1): 120-123.

Mullainathan S, Thaler RH. Behavioral Economics. Accessed November 2006 at: http://introduction.behaviouralfinance.net/MuTh.pdf.

Mullaney, TJ. October 31, 2005. This Man Wants to Heal Health Care. *Business Weekly* 3957, p 74.

Murphy v Board of Med. Examiners, 949 P.2d 530 (Ariz. Ct. App. 1997).

Naisbitt J. 1982. Megatrends. Warner Books: New York.

Neale, Ben. 2018. "Letter to State Medicaid Directors," dated January 11, 2018. Department of Health and Human Services.

Neilsen DM. 2004. What Crosby says. One of four essays on Can the gurus' concepts cure healthcare? In *Quality Progress* September pp. 26-27.

Nelson, Dave. October 2005. Baldrige—Just What the Doctor Ordered. *Quality Progress*, pp 69-75.

Neuhauser PC. 1999. Strategies for changing your corporate culture." [Re: *Frontiers of Health Services Management* Fall; 16(1): 3-29] *Frontiers of Health Services Management* 16:33-7.

Neumann E. 1955. The Great Mother: An analysis of archetype. Princeton, NJ: Princeton University Press.

NICE Manuals: Guide to the Methods of the Technology Appraisal. Accessed March 16, 2007 at: www.nice.org.uk.

Ocasio W, Kim H. 1999. The circulation of corporate control: Selection of functional backgrounds of new CEOs in large US manufacturing firms. *Administrative Science Quarterly* 44(3): 532-563.

O'Connell C. 1999. A culture of change or a change of culture? *Nursing Administration Quarterly* 23:65-8.

O'Connor JP, Nash DB, Buehler ML, Bard M. 2002. Satisfaction higher for physician executives who treat patients, survey says. *The Physician Executive* May-June pp. 16-21.

O'Daniell EE. 1999. Energizing corporate culture and creating competitive advantage: a new look at workforce programs. *Benefits Quarterly* 15:18-25.

Ogbrun PL, Julian TM, Brooker DC, et al. 1988. Perinatal Medical Negligence Closed Claims from the St. Paul Company, 1980-1982. *Journal of Reproductive Medicine* 33: 608-611.

Olasky, Marvin. 1992. The Tragedy of American Compassion. Regnery Publishers: Washington, D.C.

O'leary, DS. 1988. Will a New Federal Climate Affect Joint Commission Confidentially Policy? *Joint Commission Perspectives* Septembre/Octobre 8. 9-10: 2-4.

Oliva R. 2002. Tradeoffs in response to work pressure in the service industry. *IEEE Engineering Management Review* First Quarter pp. 53-62.

Oliver WW. Kicking the Malpractice Tort Out of Court. *Wall Street Journal*, March 19, 2013. Available at: http://online.wsj.com/article/SB10001424127887323869604578366770324716616.html.

Oostrom Tamar, Einav, Liran, Finkelstein, Amy. 2017. Outpatient Office Wait Times and Quality Of Care For Medicaid Patients. *Health Affairs* 36, no. 5 (2017): 826-832.

Orentlicher D. 2000. Medical Malpractice: Treating the Causes Instead of the Symptoms. *Medical Care* 38: 247-249.

Orlando Sentinel, April 26, 1998. Doctor's Victory Revives Proponents of Quality Care, p. A-21.

Orlando Gen. Hospital v Department of Health and Rehabilitative Servs., 567 So. 2d 962, 965 (Fla Dist. Ct. Appl. 1990).

Osnos E. September 28, 2005. In China, health care is scalpers, lines, debt. *Chicago Tribune*, Section 1, pp 1 & 6.

Owen H. Winter 1991. Learning as Transformation. The Learning Revolution (IC#27) by the Context Institute. Page 42. www.context.org/ICLIB/IC27/Owen.htm. Accessed December 2004.

Pascale RT, Sternin J. 2005. Your Company's Secret Change Agents. *Harvard Business Rev.* 83(5): 73-81.

Pathman DE, Williams ES, Konrad TR. 1996. Rural physician satisfaction: its sources and relation to retention." *Journal of Rural Health* 12(5): 366-377.

Pathman DE, Konrad TR, Williams ES, et al. 2002. Physician job satisfaction, dissatisfaction, and turnover. *Journal of Family Practice* 51:593.

Patterson KJ and Wilkins AL. You Can't Get There from Here: What Will Make Culture-Change Projects Fail, pages 262-291. In: Kilmann RH, Saxton MJ, Serpa R, et al (1985) Gaining Control of the Corporate Culture. San Francisco: Jossey-Bass.

Payne, J. April 9, 2007. Poor Getting Brushoff for Care. *Albuquerque Journal*, P. C1.

Pearson SD, Rawlins, MD. November 23/30, 2005. Quality, Innovation, and Value for Money: NICE and the British National Health Service. *JAMA* 294(20): 2618-2622.

Peirce JC. 2000. The paradox of physicians and administrators in health care organizations. *Health Care Management Review* 2(1): 7-28.

Peters TJ, Waterman RH. 1982. In Search of Excellence. Warner Books, New York, NY.

Petrock F. 1990. Corporate culture enhances profits. *HR Magazine* 35:64-6.

Pettigrew A. 1979. On Studying Organizational Culture. *Administration Science Quarterly* 24:570-81.

Pettigrew A, Ferlie E, McKee L. 1992. Shaping Strategic Change- Making change in large organizations. The Case of the National Health Service. Sage Publ., London

Pfeffer J. April 1976. Beyond management and the worker: The Institutional Function of Management. *Academy of Management Review* 1(2): 36-46.

Pfeffer J. 1994. Competitive Advantage Through People. Harvard Business School Press: Boston.

Pfeffer J, Sutton RI. 2000. The Knowing-Doing Gap. Harvard Business School Press, Boston, MA.

Phibbs CS, Bronstein JM, Buxton E, Phibbs RH. 1996. The Effects of Patient Volume and Level of Care at the Hospital of Birth on Neonatal Mortality. *Journal of the American Medical Association* 276: 1054–59.

Phillips RI. 1974. The informal organization in your hospital. *Radiologic Technology* 46(2): 101-106.

Phillips K. August 16, 2005. Hospitals increasing tapping female executives. *Nursezone.com*. At: http://nursezone.com/include/PrintArticle.asp?articleid=12529.

Pies R. March 13. 2100. Health Care is a Basic Human Right-- Almost Everywhere but Here. *OpEdNews*. Accessed March 14, 2011 at: http://www.opednews.com/articles/Health-Care-is-a-Basic-Hum-by-Ronald-Pies-110313-363.html.

Porter LW, Steers RM, Mowday RT. 1974. Organizational commitment, job satisfaction, and turnover among psychiatric technicians. *Journal of Applied Psychology* 59(5): 603-609.

Porter ME, Teisberg EO. 2006. *Redefining Health Care—Creating Value-Based Competition on Results*. Harvard Business School Publishing, Boston, MA.

Posner KL, Caplan RA, Cheney FW. 1996. Variation in Expert Opinion in Medical Malpractice Review. *Anesthesiology* 85: 1049-1054.

Potetz L, Cubanski J, Neumen. February 2011. Medicare Spending and Financing, Kaiser Family Foundation.

Prescott PA. 1986. Vacancy, stability, and turnover of registered nurses in hospitals. *Research in Nursing & Health* 9: 51-60.

Price JL, Mueller CW. 1981. A causal model of turnover for nurses. *Academy of Management Journal* 24(3): 543-565.

Pritchard RD, Campbell KM, Campbell DJ. 1977. Effects of extrinsic financial rewards on intrinsic motivation. *Journal of Applied Psychology* 62(1): 9-15.

Proenca EJ. 1996. Market orientation and organizational culture in hospitals. *Journal of Hospital Marketing* 11:3-18.

Prosser WP, Dobbs DB, Keeton RE, Owen DG. 1984. Prosser and Keeton on The Law of Torts, Fifth Edition, West Publishing Co: St Paul, MN.

Provan KG. July 1984. Interorganizational cooperation and decision making autonomy in a consortium multi-hospital system. *Academy of Management Review* 9(3): 494-504.

Public Law 89-97. 1965. "Hospital Insurance Program." [Medicaid]

Public Law 104–193. 1996. "Personal Responsibility and Work Opportunity Reconciliation Act" enacted by 104th United States Congress.

Public testimony on July 25, 2017 before the Texas Legislature, House Committee on Appropriations regarding adequacy of services provided by Texas Medicaid.

Putkowski D. 2009. Universal Coverage. Hawser Press: Media, PA.

Quam L, Dingwall R, Fenn P. 1987. Medicine and the Law, Medical Malpractice in Perspective: I—The American Experience. *British Medical Journal* 294: 1529-1532.

Quigley W. December 17, 2001. London Report: Medical missteps compound in child's death. *Albuquerque Journal*, p A2

Quigley W. October 28, 2002. The health of health care. Quoting Martin Hickey, former Lovelace CEO. *Albuquerque Journal*, Outlook, pp. 3, 9.

Quinn RE, Spreitzer GM. 1991. The Psychometrics of the competing values culture instrument and an analysis of the impact of organizational culture on quality of life. *Research in Organizational Change and Development*, 5:115-142.

Rabinowitz S, Hall DT. 1977. Organizational research on job involvement. *Psych Bull* 84:265-288.

Rand A. 1957. Atlas Shrugged. Signet books: New York.

Rasmussen, Tom. 29 July 2005. A Mandated Burden. The Wall Street Journal A-13.

Reinhardt UE. May 18, 2011. Would privatizing Medicare lead to better cost controls? *New York Times Online* accessed at: http://economix.blogs.nytimes.com/author/uwe-e-reinhardt.

Reno R. 2001. Health-care system is beyond repair. *Albuquerque Journal*, August 20. A8.

Report to Congress: Improving Incentives in the Medicare Program, June 2009. Medicare Payment Advisory Commission, Washington, DC.

Rentsch JR. 1990. Climate and culture: Interactions and qualitative differences in organizational meanings. *Journal of Applied Psychology*, 75, 668-681.

Richards BC, Thomasson G. 1992. Closed Liability Claims Analysis and the Medical Record. *Obstetrics & Gynecology* 80: 313-316.

Rickles D, Hawe P, Shiell A. 2007. A Simple guide to chaos and complexity. *Journal of Epidemiology and Community Health* 61: 933-937, accessed November 20 2007 at: doi:10.1136/jech.2006.054254.

Riter RN. 1994. Changing organizational culture. *Journal of Long-term Care Administration* 22:11-13.

Roberts G. 11/23/05. Overweight patients to be denied NHS hip operations. *London Times*, Page 2.

Robinson s. 1981. Off the Wall at Callahan's. Tor Books, NY. Page 36.

Rogers EM. 1983. Diffusion of Innovation. The Free Press, New York.

Rosch E, Lloyd BB [eds.] (1978) Cognition and Categorization. Hillsdale, N.J.: Lawrence Erlbaum.

Rothermel RC. May 1993. Mann Gulch Fire: A Race That Couldn't Be Won. *U.S. Forest Service – Rocky Mountain Research Station*. Accessed March 2006 at: http://www.fs.fed.us/rm/pubs/int_gtr299.

Rousseau L. 1984. What are the real costs of employee turnover? *CA Magazine* (Toronto) 117(2): 48-55.

Rowe, Kyle, Whitney Rowe, Josh Umbehr, Frank Dong, and Elizabeth Ablah. 2017. "Direct Primary Care in 2015: A Survey with Selected Comparisons to 2005 Survey Data." *Kansas Journal of Medicine* 10(1): 3-6.

Rowley TJ. 1997. Moving beyond dyadic ties: A network theory of stakeholder influences. *Academy of Management Review*. 22: 887-910.

Roy, Avik. July 17, 2010. UVa Study: Surgical Patients on Medicaid Are 13% More Likely to Die Than Those Without Insurance. *National Review*.

Rubin, Rita. May 2, 2018. "Is Direct Primary Care a Game Changer?" *J Amer Med Assoc.*

Rucci AJ, Kirn SP, Quinn RT. 1998. The employee-customer-profit chain at Sears. *Harvard Business Review* Jan/Feb, 83-97.

Sackett DL, Rosenberg WM, Gray JA, Haynes RB, Richardson WS. 1996. Evidence based medicine: what it is and what it isn't. *British Medical Journal* 312(7023): 71-2.

Sales, AL, Mirvis PH. 1984. When cultures collide: Issues in acquisition, in Managing Organizational Transitions by JR Kennedy, Publ: RD Irwin, Homewood, IL. pp. 107-133.

Sapienza AM: "Believing Is Seeing: How Culture Influences the Decisions Top Managers Make" pages 66-83. In: Kilmann RH, Saxton MJ, Serpa R, et al (1985) Gaining Control of the Corporate Culture. San Francisco: Jossey-Bass.

Sathe V: "How to Decipher and Change Corporate Culture" pages 230-261. In: Kilmann RH, Saxton MJ, Serpa R, et al (1985) Gaining Control of the Corporate Culture. San Francisco: Jossey-Bass.

Schein EH: "How culture forms, develops and changes," pages 17-43. In: Kilmann RH, Saxton MJ, Serpa R, et al (1985) Gaining Control of the Corporate Culture. San Francisco: Jossey-Bass.

Schelling TC. 1960. The Strategy of Conflict. Cambridge: Harvard University Press.

Schneider J. 1976. The "greener grass" phenomenon: Differential effects of a work context alternative on organizational participation and withdrawal intentions. *Organizational Behavior and Human Performance* 16: 308-33.

Schwartz WB, Komesar NK. 1978. Doctors, Damages and Deterrence. *New England Journal of Medicine* 298: 1282-1289.

Schyve PM. 2004. What Feigenbaum says. One of four essays on "Can the gurus' concepts cure healthcare?" *Quality Progress* September pp. 30-33.

Scott RA, Aiken LH, Mechanic D, Moravcsik J. 1995. Organizational aspects of caring. *Millbank Quarterly* 73(1): 77-95

Scott T, Mannion R, Davies H, Marshall M. 2003. The Quantitative Measurement of Organizational Culture in Health Care: A Review of the Available Instruments. *Health Services Research* 38(3): 923-38.

Seago J. 1997. Organizational Culture in Hospitals: Issues in Measurement. *Journal of Nursing Measurement* 5 (2): 165-78.

Senge PM. 1990. The Fifth Discipline-The Art and Practice of the Learning Organization. Currency Doubleday, New York.

Sfikas PM. 1998. Are Insurers Making Treatment Decisions? *JADA* 129: 1036-1039.

Shader K, Broome ME, Broome CD, et al. April 2001. Factors influencing satisfaction and anticipated turnover for nurses at an academic medical center. *Journal of Nursing Administration* 31(4): 210-216.

Shanahan MM. 1993. A comparative analysis of recruitment and retention of health care professionals. *Health Care Management Review* 18(3): 41-51.

Shanks H (1968) *The Art and Craft of Judging—The Decision of Learned Hand.* Macmillan Co., New York.

Shannon v. McNulty, M.D., 718 A.2d 828, (S.Ct.Pa. 1998) and Corporate Health Insurance, Inc. v. Texas Department of

Insurance, 215 F.3d 526 (5thCir.2000) (rehearing den'd, 2000 WL 1035524) and Tex Civ. Prac. & Rem., § 88.001 et seq.; Tex. Ins. Code, art. 20A.09(e), 20A.12(a & b); 20A.12A, 28. 58A § 6(b & c), 28.58A § 6A, 21.58A § 8(f), 21.58C.

Shaw GB. 1913. Preface to The Doctor's Dilemma, Penguin: Baltimore. Reprinted in 1954.

Sheikh A, Hurwitz B. 1999. A national database of medical errors. *Journal of the Royal Society of Medicine* November 92: 554-555.

Sheikh, K. 2003. Reliability of provider volume and outcome associations for healthcare policy. *Medical Care* October, 41(10): 1111-1117.

Sherer JL. 1994. Corporate cultures. Turning 'us versus them' into 'we.'" *Hospitals & Health Networks* 68:20-2, 24, 26-7.

Shortell SM. Fall 1988. The evolution of hospital systems: Unfulfilled promises and self-fulfilling prophecies. *Medical Care Review* 45: 745-772.

Shortell SM, Gillies RR, Anderson DA, Mitchell JB, Morgan KL. Winter 1993. Creating organized delivery systems: The barriers and facilitators. *Hospital & Health Services Administration* 38(4): 447-466.

Shortell SM, O'Brien JL, Carman JM, et al. June 1995. Assessing the impact of continuous quality improvement/total quality management: Concept versus implementation. *Health Services Research* 30(2): 377-401.

Shortell S. March 1997. Commentary on: "Physician-Hospital integration and the economic theory of the firm" by JC Robinson. *Medical Care Research and Review* 54:3-24.

Shortell SM, Bennett CL, Byck GR. 1998. Assessing the impact of continuous quality improvement on clinical practice: What it will take to accelerate progress. *Millbank Quarterly* 76(4): 593-624.

Shortell S, Waters T, Budetti P, Clarke K. 1998. Physicians as double agents: Maintaining trust in an era of multiple accountabilities. *JAMA* 23: 1102-1108.

Shortell SM, Gillies RR, Anderson DA, Morgan-Erickson K, Mitchell J. 2000. Remaking Health Care in America: The Evolution of Organized Delivery Systems. San Francisco: Jossey-Bass.

Shortell SM, Jones RH, Rademaker AW, et al. 2000. Assessing the Impact of Total Quality management and Organizational Culture on Multiple Outcomes of Care for Coronary Artery Bypass Graft Surgery Patients. *Medical Care* 38 (2): 207-17.

Shortell SM, Zazzali JL, Burns LR, et al. 2001. Implementing Evidence-Based Medicine: The Role of Market Pressures, Compensation Incentives, and Culture in Physician Organization. *Medical Care* 39 (7, Supplement): I-62-78.

Shorter E. 1985. Bedside Manners. Simon & Schuster: New York

Sieveking N, Bellet W, Marston RC. 1993. Employees' view of their work experience in private hospitals. *Health Services Management Research* 6 (2): 129-38.

Simone JV. 1999. Understanding Academic Medical Centers: Simone's Maxims. *Clinical Cancer Research* 5:2281-2285.

Simunovic M, To T, Theriault, M, et al. Pediatric Cardiac Surgery: The Effect of Hospital and Surgeon Volume on In-hospital Mortality. *Pediatrics* 1998; 101(6): 963-69.

Simons R, Davila A. 1998. "How high is your return on management? *Harvard Business Review* 76; 70-80

Smircich, L. 1985. Is the concept of culture a paradigm for understanding organizations and ourselves? In P. J. Frost, L. F. Moore, M. R. Louis, C. C. Lundberg, and J. Martin (Eds.), Organizational Culture (pp. 55-72). Beverly Hills, Calif.: Sage.

Smith B, West K. 2002. Death certification: an audit of practice entering the 21st century. *Journal of Clinical Pathology* 55: 275-279.

Smith GCS, Pell JP. 2003. Parachute use to prevent death and major trauma related to gravitational challenge: systematic review of randomized controlled trials. *British Medical Journal* 327: 1459-61.

Smith GP. 2008. Accessing health care resources: Economic, Medical, Ethical and Socio-legal challenges. In: Weisstub DN, Diaz Pintos G. Autonomy and Human Rights in Health Care. Springer: The Netherlands.

Smith FJ. 1977. Work attitudes as predictors of attendance on a specific day. *Journal of Applied Psychology* 62(1): 16-19.

Smith HL, Yourstone S, Lorber D, Mann B. 2001. Managed care and medical practice guidelines: The thorny problem of attaining physician compliance. In Advances in Health Care Management, Vol II, Elsevier Science Ltd., New York, NY.

Smith HL, Waldman JD, Fottler M, Hood JN. 2005. Chapter 5: Strategic Management of Internal Customers: Building Value through Human Capital and Culture; Advances in Health Care Management, Volume 6: Strategic Thinking and Entrepreneurial Action in the Health Care Industry. Emerald Insight: Bingley, West Yorkshire, England.

Soffel D, Luft HS. 1993. Anatomy of health care reform proposals. *Western Journal of Medicine* 159: 494-500.

Spear S, Bowen HK. 1999. Decoding the DNA of the Toyota Production system. *Harvard Business Review* September/October pp. 97-106.

Spear SJ. September 2005. Fixing Healthcare from the Inside, Today. *Harvard Business Review,* pp. 2-16.

Steel RP, Ovalle NK. 1984. A Review and meta-analysis of research on the relationship between behavioral intentions and employee turnover. *Journal of Applied Psychology* 69(4): 673-686.

Steiger B. Nov/Dec 2006. Survey Results: Doctors Say Morale Is Hurting. *Physician Executive.* Pp. 6-15. Accessed January 23, 2006 at: www.acpe.org/education/surveys/morale/morale.htm.

Sterman JD. 2002. Systems dynamics modeling: Tools for learning in a complex world. *IEEEE Engineering Management Review* First Quarter pp. 42-52.

Sterman J. 2006. Learning from evidence on a complex world. *American Journal of Public Health* 96: 505-514.

Stevenson, K. 2000. Are your Practices Resistant to Changing Their Clinical Culture? *Primary Care Report* 2 (5): 19-20.

Stocking B. 1992. Promoting change in clinical care. *Quality in health care* 1: 56-60.

Stoller JK, Orens DK, Kester L. March 2001. The impact of turnover among respiratory care practitioners in a health care system: Frequency and associated costs. *Respiratory Care* 46(3): 238-242.

Stossel T, Shaywitz D. July 9, 2006. Biotech Bucks Don't Corrupt Researchers. Reprinted from the *Washington Post* in the *Albuquerque Journal*, Page B3.

Stout, MK. March 2006. Medicaid: Yesterday, Today and Tomorrow—A short history of Medicaid Policy and its impact on Texas. Texas Public Policy Foundation.

Stowe JD. 2000. Staff turnover or staff retention: Understanding the dynamics of generations at work in the 21st century. *Canadian Veterinary Journal* 41(10): 803-808.

Strawn, Julie, Mark Greenberg, and Steve Savner. 2001. *Improving Employment Outcomes Under TANF.* Center for Law and Social Policy.

Stross, C. 2004. The Family Trade. Tom Doherty Associates Books: New York.

Stubblefield A. 2005. The Baptist Healthcare Journey to Excellence, Wiley & Sons: Hoboken, NJ.

Studdert DM, Thomas EJ, Burstin HR, Orav J, Brennan TA. 2000. Negligent Care and Malpractice Claiming Behavior in Utah and Colorado. *Medical Care* 38: 250-260.

Studer, Q. 2003. Hardwiring Excellence. Gulf Breeze, FL. Fire Starter Publishing

Surowiecki J. 2004. The Wisdom of Crowds. Anchor Books: New York.

Swift B, West K. 2002. Death certification: an audit of practice entering the 21st century. *Journal of Clinical Pathology* 55: 275-279.

Tai TWC, Bame SI, Robinson CD. 1998. Review of nursing turnover research, 1977-1996. *Society of Science in Medicine.* 47(12): 1905-1924.

Tallahassee Mem'l Reg'l Med. Ctr. v. Cook, 109 F.3d 693 (11th Cir. 1997).

Taragin MI, Wilczek AP, Karns ME, Trout R, Carson JL. 1992. Physician demographics and the risk of medical malpractice. *American Journal of Medicine* 93: 537-542.

Taragin MI, Sonnenberg FA, Karns ME, Trout R, Shapiro S, Carson JL. 1994. Does Physician Performance Explain Interspecialty Differences in Malpractice Claim Rates? *Medical Care* 32: 661-667.

Tate, NJ. 2012. Obamacare Survival Guide. Humanix Books: West Palm Beach, FL.

Testimony of the public before Texas legislature on July 25, 2017.

Texas Government Code. 2011. Medicaid Reform Waiver, Title 4, Subtitle I, Chapter 537.

TMA (Texas Medical Association). 2017. "TMA Survey Results, 2017 and Preus years."

Thomas C, Ward M, Chorba C, Kumiega A. 1990. Measuring and interpreting organizational culture. *Journal of Nursing Administration* 20(6): 17-24.

Thomas EJ, Studdert DM, Burstin HR, et al. 2000. Incidence and Types of Adverse Events and Negligent Care in Utah and Colorado. *Medical Care* 38: 261-271.

Thompson, Clive. December 10, 2006. Bicycle Helmets Put You at Risk. *The New York Times Magazine*, Section 6, Page 36.

TMA, 2016. Survey of Texas Physicians, 2016. Texas Medical Association.

Tribus M. 1992. The germ theory of management. *National Institute for Engineering Management & Systems,* Publication #1459

Tribus M. February 1992. Reducing Deming's 14 Points to practice. *Quality First.* National Institute for Engineering Management and Systems, NSPE Publication #1459

Trice HM, Beyer JM (1984) "Studying organizational cultures through rites and ceremonials." *Academy of Management Review* 9(4): 653-669.

Trigg B. February 25, 2011. Make Health Care A Right for All. *Albuquerque Journal*, A9.

Tucker R, McCoy W, Evans. 1990. Can questionnaires Objectively Assess Organizational Culture? *Journal of Managerial Psychology* 5 (4): 4-11.

Tuchman B. 1984. The March of Folly. Alfred Knopf: New York.

US General Accounting Office (GAO). Impact on Hospital and Physician Costs Extends Beyond Insurance. *Medical Liability* 95.169 (1995): 1-17.

Uttal B. October 17, 1983. The Corporate Culture Vultures. *Fortune* pp. 66-72.

Van der Merwe R, Miller S. 1971. The Measurement of Labour Turnover. *Human Relations* 24(3): 233-253.

Van Watson GH. 2002. Peter F. Drucker: Delivering Value to Customers. *Quality Progress* May pp. 55-61.

Vergara GH. 1999. Finding a compatible corporate culture. *Healthcare Executive* 14:46-7.

Verma, Seema. "Seema Verma to Jon Hamdorf." May 7, 2018.

Veterans Health Administration, September 2015. "Review of Alleged Mismanagement at the Health Eligibility Center." *Office of the Inspector General.*

Vitkine B. 2012. Inside the dramatic collapse of Greece's healthcare system. Accessed December 2012 at: http://www.businessinsider.com/collapse-of-greeces-healthcare-system-2012-12.

Waldman JD, Young TS, Pappelbaum SJ, Turner SW, Kirkpatrick SE, George L. 1982. Pediatric cardiac catheterization with 'same-day' discharge. *American Journal of Cardiology* 50:800-804.

Waldman JD, Pappelbaum SJ, George L, et al. 1984. Cost-containment strategies in congenital heart disease. *Western Journal of Medicine* 141:123-126.

Waldman JD, Ratzan RM, Pappelbaum SJ. 1998. Physicians must abandon the *illusion* of autonomy.... *Pediatric Cardiology* 19:9-17.

Waldman JD. 2001. Aim with Echo in Pulmonary Atresia (The echo machine *works* in the cath lab.) *Pediatric Cardiology* 22(2): 91-92.

Waldman JD, McCullough G. 2002. A Calculus of *Unnecessary* Echocardiograms—Application of management principles to healthcare. *Pediatric Cardiology* 23: 186-191.

Waldman JD, Spector RA. 2003. Malpractice claims analysis yields widely applicable principles. *Pediatric Cardiology* 24(2): 109-117.

Waldman JD, Smith HL, Hood JN. 2003. Corporate Culture — The missing piece of the healthcare puzzle. *Hospital Topics* 81(1): 5-14.

Waldman JD, Schargel F. 2003. Twins in Trouble: The need for system-wide reform of both Healthcare and Education. *Total*

Quality Management & Business Excellence, October 14(8): 895-901.

Waldman JD, Yourstone SA, Smith HL. 2003. Learning Curves in Healthcare. *Health Care Management Review* 28(1): 43-56.

Waldman, JD, Smith HL, Kelly F, Arora S. 2004. The Shocking Cost of Turnover in Healthcare. *Health Care Management Review* 29(1): 2-7.

Waldman JD, Arora S. 2004. Retention rather than turnover—A Better and Complementary HR Method. *Human Resource Planning* 27(3): 6-9.

Waldman JD, Hood JN, Smith HL, et al. 2004. Changing the Approach to Workforce Movements: Application of Net Retention Rate. *Journal of Applied Business and Economics.* 24(2): 38-60.

Waldman JD, Schargel F. 2006. Twins in Trouble (II): Systems Thinking in Healthcare and Education. *Total Quality Management & Business Excellence* 17(1): 117-130.

Waldman JD, Arora S, Smith HL, Hood JN. 2006. Improving medical practice outcomes by retaining clinicians. *Journal of Medical Practice Management* March/April pp. 263-271.

Waldman JD. 2006. Change the Metrics: If *you get what you measure,* then measure what you want—retention." *Journal of Medical Practice Management* July/August, pp. 1-7.

Waldman JD, Hood JN, Smith HL. 2006. Healthcare CEO and Physician—Reaching Common Ground. *Journal of Healthcare Management.* May/June 51(3): 171-187.

Waldman JD, Yourstone SA, Smith HL. 2007. Learning-*The* Means to Improve Medical Outcomes. *Health Services Management Research* 2007; 20: 227-237.

Waldman JD, Smith HL. 2007. Thinking Systems need Systems Thinking. *Systems Research and Behavioral Science* 24: 1-15.

Waldman JD, Cohn K. September 2007. Mend the *Gap*. In The Business of Health, Editors: KH Cohn & D Hough, Praeger Perspectives, New York.

Waldman JD. 2009. The Triple Standard in Healthcare. *California Journal of Politics & Policy* 1(1): 1-13.

Waldman JD. 2010. Uproot US Healthcare. ADM Books: Albuquerque, NM.

Waldman JD. 2010. Cambio Radical al Sistema de Salud de los Estados Unidos. ADM Books: Albuquerque, NM.

Waldman, Deane. 2013. THE HEALTH OF HEALTHCARE (I) – The Right Approach is Medical. *J Med Pract Med*, July/August, pp. 29-31. Reprinted (by request) in *Podiatry Management Magazine*.

Waldman JD. 2013. The Cancer in Healthcare – How Greed Is Killing What We Love. Hugo House Publishers: Denver, CO.

Waldman JD. 2013. THE HEALTH OF HEALTHCARE (II) – Healthcare Has Cancer. *Journal of Medical Practice Management* Sept/Oct Pages 113-116.

Waldman JD. 2013. THE HEALTH OF HEALTHCARE (III) – Dissolving (Curing) the Cancer in Healthcare. *Journal of Medical Practice Management* Nov/Dec, Pages 184-186.

Waldman JD. March 2014. The U.S. Needs Tort Replacement, Not Just 'Reform.' *Journal of Socialomics* 3:107. doi: 10.4172/2167-0358.1000107.

Waldman JD. 2014. THE HEALTH OF HEALTHCARE (V) – Is the Very Freedom of Providers At Risk? *J Med Pract Med,* May/June, Vol. 29, No. 6, Pp. 366-368.

Waldman JD. 2014. THE HEALTH OF HEALTHCARE (VI) – Be Prepared! *Journal of Medical Practice Management* July/August, Pp. 64-66.

Waldman JD. November 2015. The Cancer in the American Healthcare System – How Washington Controls and

Destroys Our Health Care. Strategic Book Publishing & Rights Agency: Corpus Christi, TX.

Waldman JD. December 21, 2015. Bureaucracy, not drugs, drives health costs. *Wall Street Journal*, page A12.

Waldman, Deane. 2016. Our Allies Have Become Our Enemies. Gatekeeper Press: Columbus, Ohio.

Waldman, Deane. 2016. Washington's BARRC Is Its Bite. Gatekeeper Press: Columbus, Ohio.

Waldman, Deane. 2016. The Root Cause That Washington Conceals. Gatekeeper Press: Columbus, Ohio.

Waldman, Deane. 2016. Is Obamacare the Answer? Gatekeeper Press: Columbus, Ohio.

Waldman, Deane. 2016. Government Hypocrisy over Epipen: The Pot Calling the Kettle Black. *Forbes*.

Waldman, Deane. 2016. Single Payer Won't Save Us. Gatekeeper Press: Columbus, Ohio.

Waldman, Deane. November 12, 2016. The Great Disruptor Can Fix Healthcare. *The Hill*.

Waldman, Deane. December 5, 2016. Obamacare's Dangerous Wait Lines. *The Hill*.

Waldman, Deane. December 14, 2017. Healthcare Regulations are Hazardous to your Health. *The Hill*.

Waldman, Deane. January 4, 2017. A doctor's straight talk: America, your health care is not a federal responsibility. *Fox News*.

Waldman, Deane. January 10, 2017. California wants single payer and Texas wants free market — say hello to 'StatesCare.' *The Hill*.

Waldman, Deane. March 2017. The Saga of 1115—A Waiver Can Fix Texas Medicaid, But Only Temporarily. Texas Public Policy Foundation

Waldman, Deane. May 8, 2017. Administrative job growth in healthcare isn't good for America. *The Hill*.

Waldman, Deane. May 23, 2017. More coverage doesn't necessarily translate into better patient care. *The Hill*.

Waldman, Deane, Ginn, Vance. June14, 2017. California and Texas Agree on Health Care. *Real Clear Health*.

Waldman, Deane. September 25, 2017. Think Obamacare Is Bad? 'Medicare for All' Would Make Things Even Worse. *Daily Signal*.

Waldman, Deane. 2018. The Cure for U.S. Healthcare–*StatesCare* and the Texas Model. Gatekeeper Press: Columbus, Ohio.

Waldman, Deane. February 8, 2018. Americans can be entitled or free — but not both. *The Hill*.

Waldman, Deane. March 8, 2018. Texas deserves credit for running health care the right way. *The Hill*.

Waldman, Deane. May 10, 2018. Great Britain Offers Cautionary Tale on Single Payer. *Real Clear Health*.

Waldman, Deane. June 28, 2018. Conflating Health Insurance with Health Care. *Real Clear Health*.

Waldman, Deane. July 28, 2018. Medicare for All is a socialist's dream — and an American Nightmare. *The Hill*.

Walker J, Pan Eric, Douglas J, Adler-Milstein J, Bates DW, Middleton B. January 2005. The Value of Health Care Information Exchange and Interoperability. *Health Affairs*. W 5—10-18.

Wall Street Journal Editorial, January 2, 2003. Lawyers vs. Patients---III, p. A14.

Wall Street Journal Online. May 10, 2011. National Health Preview: RomneyCare's bad outcomes keep coming.

Wallach EJ. 1983. Individuals and organizations: The cultural match. *Training and Development Journal* 37: 29-36.

Walshe K, Rundall TG. 2001. Evidence-based management: From theory to practice in health care. *Millbank Quarterly*, 79(3): 429-457.

Ward, Bryce, and Brandon Bridge. 2018. *The Economic Impact of Medicaid Expansion in Montana.* University of Montana Bureau of Business and Economic Research.

Ward CJ. 1991. Analysis of 500 obstetric and gynecologic malpractice claims: Causes and prevention. *American Journal of Obstetrics and Gynecology,* 165: 298306.

Watts, AW. 1951. The Wisdom of Insecurity. Pantheon Books: New York.

Watson GH. 2002. Peter F. Drucker. Delivering Value to Customers. *Quality Progress,* May pp. 55-61.

Weber J, Wheelwright S. 1997. Massachusetts General Hospital: CABG Surgery (A). *Harvard Business School Case,* # 9-696-015.

Weick KE. 1993. The collapse of sensemaking in organizations: The Mann Gulch Disaster. *Administrative Science Quarterly* 38: 628-652.

Weil TP. 1987. The changing relationship between physicians and the hospital CEO. *Trustee,* Feb; 40(2): 15-18.

Weil PA. 1990. Job turnover of CEOs in teaching and nonteaching hospitals. *Academic Med,* 65(1): 1-7.

Weisman CS, Alexander CS, Chase GA. 1981. Determinants of hospital staff nurse turnover. *Medical Care* 19(4): 431-443.

Wickline v. State, 192 Cal. App.3d 16.0.1645 (1986), 239 Cal. Rptr. 805,825.

Wicks E. 2007. Human Rights and Healthcare. Hart Publishing: Portland, OR.

Wiener, Y. 1988. Forms of value systems: A focus on organizational effective-ness, cultural change, and maintenance. *Academy of Management Review* 13: 534-545.

Wilcox FK. 1993. Corporate culture in a mythless society. *American Journal of Medical Quality* 1993; 8: 134-7.

Wilson CN, Meadors AC. 1990. Hospital Chief Executive Officer Turnover. *Hospital Topics* 68(1): 35-39.

Wilson CN, Stranahan H. 2000. Organizational characteristics associated with hospital CEO turnover. *Journal of Health Care Management* 45(6): 395-404.

Wilson L. July 22, 2004. Healthier habits will reduce medical costs. *Albuquerque Journal* A13.

Winton R, March 18, 2009. Former City of Angels hospital executive pleads guilty to paying kickbacks. Accessed March 2009 at: http://latimes.com/news/local/la-me-medfraud19-2009mar19,0,934741.story.

Wise LC. 1990. Tracking turnover. *Nursing Economic$* 8(1): 45-51

Wittkower ED, Stauble WJ. 1972. Psychiatry and the general practitioner. *Psychiatry Med* 3:287-301.

Wood KM, Matthews GE. 1997. Overcoming the physician group-hospital cultural gap. *Healthcare Financial Management* 51:69-70.

Woods, TE. 2009. Meltdown. Regenery Publishing: Washington, DC.

Woolhandler S, Campbell T, Himmelstein DU. 2003. Costs of Health Care Administration in the United States and Canada. *New England Journal of Medicine* 349:768-775.

Wu AW, Cavanaugh TA, McPhee SJ, Lo B, Micco GP. 1997. To tell the truth—Ethical and Practical Issues in disclosing medical mistakes to patients. *Journal of General Internal Medicine* 12: 770-775.

Wysocki B. April 9, 2004. To fix health care, hospitals take tips from factory floor. *Wall Street Journal* A6.

Yelle LE. 1979. The Learning Curve—Historical Review and Comprehensive Survey. *Decision Science* 302–28.

Yeung KO, Brockbank JW, Ulrich DO. 1991. Organizational culture and human resource practices: an empirical assessment. *Research in Organizational Change and Development* 5: 59-82.

Young GJ, Charns MP, Daley J, et al. Best Practices for Managing Surgical Services: The Role of Coordination. *Health Care Management Review* 1997; 22(4): 72-81.

Younossi, Zobair. June 3, 2018. HCV outcomes worse for patients with public insurance, Medicaid. *Digestive Disease Weekly*.

Zammuto RF, Krakower JY. 1991. Quantitative and qualitative studies of organizational culture. *Res in Organizational Change and Development* 5:83-114.

Zimmerman R, Oster C. June 24, 2002. Insurers' missteps helped provoke malpractice 'crisis.' *Wall Street Journal*, pp 1, 8.

Zoppo, Avalon, Amanda Santos, and Jackson Hudgins. October 2017. "Here's the Full List of Donald Trump's Executive Orders," *NBC News*.

Zuger, A. 2004. "Dissatisfaction with Medical Practice." *New England Journal of Medicine* 350(1): 69-76.

Dr. Deane's Healthcare Decoder

D r. Deane Waldman's Healthcare Decoder is purely functional. It takes the mystery and confusion out of healthcare and replaces them with understanding. Whether the complexity is intentional or not, the language and terms people use in healthcare are often confusing and make no sense. Sometimes they mean the opposite of what you think they mean.

This Decoder does precisely what you want it to do: it decodes. It turns healthcare gibberish into easy-to-understand language.

Healthcare versus **health care** = As one word, *healthcare* means a huge system that consumes nearly 20 percent of the U.S. annual GDP. *Health care*—two words—refers to a close personal (fiduciary) service relationship, protected by law, between a patient and a provider.

* * *

ACA = **A**ffordable **C**are **A**ct, also known colloquially as Obamacare. Keep in mind the law's full name—Patient Protection and Affordable Health Care Act of 2010 (PPAHCA)—to remember what it was supposed to do for us.

Adverse impact = where a patient is harmed during, not necessarily by, health care. This is a negative patient outcome, such as failure to improve, or being sicker or worse after treatment. Contrast this *outcome* or result to the words "error" or "mistake" that refer to a *behavior* or action, not an outcome. You can read details about the important difference between behavior and outcome in *The Cancer in the American Healthcare System.* (See Error/mistake.)

Adverse selection = when an insurance carrier has a large number of sick enrollees, who therefore require the carrier to pay large medical bills. This is "adverse," i.e., a negative result, for the insurance company's bottom line. With enough adverse selection, an insurance carrier could lose enough money paying medical claims to go bankrupt. Before this happens, a carrier will simply stop selling medical insurance as several have already done.

APTC = <u>A</u>dvanced <u>P</u>remium <u>T</u>ax <u>C</u>redit, more commonly known as "ACA subsidies." This refers to the money offered by the federal government to offset increased cost of health insurance premiums. There is a sliding scale for the amount of subsidy from 400 percent of the poverty line ($93,132 per year) to 138 percent of the poverty line ($23,283). Between 138 percent and 400 percent, you get a subsidy, but less as your income increases. Above 400 percent, there is no subsidy. Below 138 percent of the poverty line, you are eligible for free insurance through Medicaid, assuming you are a legal citizen. Under the ACA, 79 percent of the U.S. population qualifies for some amount of subsidy. Median household income in the U.S. in September 2014 was $51,939.

Balance billing = a practice where the provider bills the patient for the difference between what insurance pays and the actual charges.

BARRC = **B**ureaucracy, **A**dministration, **R**ules, **R**egulations, and **C**ompliance. Acronym that stands for what a bureaucracy is and does.

Benefit = services or items that the insurance coverage will pay for. It does not guarantee that you will actually receive the benefit, only that *if you can get* the covered care, the insurer will pay a contracted amount to the provider.

Big Pharma = a common nickname for huge, usually multinational pharmaceutical companies, such as GlaxoSmithKline, Johnson & Johnson, Merck, Pfizer, and Roche.

Bureaucracy = excessively complicated administrative process or system. For my purposes, "bureaucracy" includes (1) administration such as eligibility, confirmation, billing, coding, payment, and distribution; (2) insurance activities from actuarial analysis to authorization; and (3) the regulatory machine from rule making through the review process to compliance oversight and accreditation or loss of accreditation.

Burwell *v.* Hobby Lobby: See SCOTUS.

Butterfly effect = is a crude way of describing the Law of Disproportionate Consequences. This "law" states that small actions can have big outcomes, and conversely, grand actions can have trivial or insignificant results. As an example in healthcare, consider the massive effort and huge expense of Obamacare that produced little or no beneficial effect for We the Patients.

Cadillac Tax = is part of PPAHCA. It levies a 40 percent tax on any insurance premium that costs annually more than $10,200 for an individual or $27,500 for a family. This tax has little to do with personal income and everything to do with benefits of the insurance plan. The Cadillac Tax will hit those in high-risk occupations such as construction workers, firefighters, and police officers.

Cancer = where a previously healthy cell in a human body or part of a system no longer performs its normal functions and begins to grow uncontrollably, ultimately killing the person or the system.

CBO (contrast to GAO) = The Congressional Budget Office is tasked with predicting the *future* economic and budgetary effects of congressional action. For example, the CBO has calculated the future cost of PPAHCA as low as $1.1 trillion and as high as $1.7 trillion. (See GAO.)

CCIIO (pronounced sis-eye-oh) = The Center for Consumer Information and Insurance Oversight. CCIIO is another federal agency that creates and oversees insurance rules and compliance with healthcare regulations, specifically with the Affordable Care Act (ACA).

Charge = the price, or what you see on a Bill for Payment. This has no relationship, repeat *no relationship,* to what is actually paid or the true cost.

CLASS Act = The Community Living Assistance Services and Support Act was Title VII in the ACA. It was intended to create a voluntary, public, long-term care insurance program, but was deleted from the act by the White House seven months after the ACA was signed into law.

CMS = Centers for Medicare & Medicaid Services. This is the federal agency that funds and oversees both programs.

COBRA = Consolidated Omnibus Budget Reconciliation Act of 1985. Allows a patient to keep insurance temporarily after employment ends. The employer no longer pays any portion of the premium: the insured pays

100 percent plus an administrative fee. There are other restrictions.

Complexity = According to the dictionary, complex means "composed of many different and connected parts." It also means "not easy to understand." Complexity in healthcare comes in two forms: inherent and artificial.

Compliance over science = following the rules is more important than the patient. If a clinical guideline says one thing but the latest data or a doctor's well-honed judgment says something different, the doctor must follow the approved clinical pathway.

Concierge medicine = also called "direct-pay medicine." This refers to doctors who do not accept insurance, but rather have the patients pay them directly. This usually involves a retainer fee that covers office visits. Most direct-pay practices negotiate large discounts at labs and with hospitals as well as pharmacies, because the patients will pay cash. By cutting out the insurance carriers, these practices dramatically reduce both their administrative expenses and the time doctors now spend on bureaucratic nonsense.

Consumer = In both health care—the service, as well as healthcare—the system, the consumer is the patient. Personally, I dislike the word "consumer" as it refers to a purely one-way relationship: doctor delivers and patient consumes. We all know that good medicine is a two-way relationship, a partnership, not a delivery service.

It is important to recognize that healthcare is currently a third-party payer system, meaning the *consumer* of goods and services is not the *payer* for the goods and services consumed. She or he does not pay the supplier (provider) of services and goods—the third party does. Thus, there is micro-economic disconnection, where supply and demand—that are normally connected by supplier competition and demander's (consumer's) money—are *disconnected*. This prevents the functioning of the free-market forces. (See Micro-economic disconnection.)

CO-OP = Consumer Operated & Oriented Plan established by the ACA law. Co-ops are not-for-profit insurance companies that were given large sums of taxpayer dollars—more than $2.4 billion in low-interest loans (down from the initial $6 billion)—by the federal government to offer low-cost alternatives to insurance products sold by commercial for-profit companies. These co-ops are not co-ops in the usual sense, as the customers do not participate in profits and losses. As of June 2016, 13 of the 23 ACA-established insurance co-ops have either closed or have been declared insolvent. Nine of the remaining 10 are near insolvency. ACA co-ops are going out of business because of simple economics: they are paying out more in mandated benefits than they are taking in as revenue.

Co-pay (insurance term) = a payment you make to the doctor, typically $5–20, when you go for care. This is in addition to what the insurance company will pay the doctor on your behalf for your care services and in addition to the cost of your premiums.

Cosmology episode = a condition where the world makes no sense, where for instance, the sun rises out of the south. This is what providers of health care face every day. They think they are doing what patients want and yet the "system" in which they work obstructs, constrains, and punishes them. This makes no sense—healthcare is a cosmology episode for people who work in healthcare.

Cost = is the most misunderstood and, therefore, misused word in healthcare language. You and I use "cost" to mean the sum of all materials, labor, and capital to produce a product or service. Using that definition, no one knows the cost of anything in health care as well as healthcare. In the world of healthcare, "cost" is allocated, apportioned, back calculated, and projected, but not the simple sum of all factors of production and distribution. Be sure you understand that anyone who claims to report the true cost of anything in healthcare is guessing.

Cost-sharing reduction (CSR) = there are two forms of CSR and they are quite different. There are *patient* CSRs where the patient must pay a portion of the bill for service in addition to what was paid as a premium. There are *federal* CSRs where Congress will subsidize the expenses of an insurance company trying to reduce the premium costs that patients will pay. Federal CSRs are also known as "bailouts."

Covered life = someone who has signed up with a qualified health plan for insurance. As soon as the insurance card is issued, the person is covered for 90 days, even if that individual does not pay the premiums.

Debt versus deficit (U.S. national) = often confused, but quite different. The **deficit** is the amount the government spends per year greater than the amount the government takes in as revenue. For the past 10 years, the deficit has been approximately 30 percent, meaning if we took in $2 trillion, we spent $3 trillion. To cover the annual deficit, each year the government must borrow the amount of the deficit. This accumulated borrowing is called the national **debt**, which has increased from $7 trillion (2004) to $12 trillion (2009) to $19 trillion (2016). The 2018 national debt is approaching $21 trillion. Eventually, someone will have to pay this back. Meanwhile, the public pays debt service on the national debt. In 2015, just the service on this debt cost us $400 billion.

Deductible (insurance term) = a predetermined amount of money you must pay before your insurance company will pay your claim. This is in addition to the cost of your premiums.

Defensive medicine = when providers make decisions based on how their record will look, not necessarily on what is best for the patient.

Diagnosis = literally means "the identification of the *nature* of an illness." Nature can mean only the description of the ailment and/or it can mean the root cause of your problem. Many, in fact most, diagnoses are descriptive, not etiologic. (See Root cause.)

Dissolve (a problem) = is the most desirable of the four ways to "solve" a problem. It is described in detail in *The Cancer in the American Healthcare System*. To dissolve a problem means you change the system so the root cause of the problem no longer exists. Therefore, the problem cannot recur because the root cause is gone.

"Donut hole" = a gap in coverage in Medicare (Part D) where the beneficiary has to pay all of his or her prescription drug costs. The gap is between where the initial, minimum coverage ends, and when the beneficiary has spent enough to reach the catastrophic coverage threshold.

Down-code = use of a billing code by a health care provider to give a reduced rate for health care services or goods provided. Believe it or not, this is illegal.

Effectiveness (contrast to efficiency) = refers to how successful a person, organization, or system is in achieving the desired effect. In baseball, an effective pitcher is one who throws strikes that people cannot hit. An effective healthcare system makes and keeps the most people as healthy and as long-lived as possible. *An effective system is always efficient, but an efficient one may not be effective.*

Efficiency (contrast to effectiveness) = is classically defined in terms of work per unit time, but it really means using the least resources (money, labor, power) while working. You can be very efficient and still be ineffective. If you can produce 10 buggy whips per hour but nobody wants to buy them, you are highly efficient but not effective (at producing income for your company). In healthcare, if you see 10 patients per hour, you are very efficient. If they all remain ill, you are NOT effective.

EHB = Essential Health Benefits. This is a federally mandated list of health services that an insurance plan must offer in order to be compliant with the ACA.

Employer mandate = law that requires businesses with 50 or more full-time employees to provide health insurance to at least 95 percent of their employees and dependents up to age 26. If they don't, employers have to pay some steep fees, which can be as high as $2,000 per month per uninsured employee.

EMR = Electronic Medical Record. This system converts hard copy records and prescriptions to digital format. As users, doctors and nurses find EMR quite *un*friendly; it is overly cumbersome, excessively time-consuming, and extreme costly. Time required to utilize EMR is time the provider cannot spend with the patient or researching the case.

EMTALA = Emergency Medical Treatment and Labor Act of 1986, also known as the "anti-dumping law." This requires emergency rooms to care for (rather than transfer) any acutely, seriously ill patient, regardless of whether the patient has any payment source or not. EMTALA created the *unfunded mandate.*

Enrollment period (for buying insurance) — a limited amount of time, usually two–three months, when you are allowed to buy or make changes to your health insurance. The rest of the year you cannot purchase government-supported health insurance.

Entitlement = a legal right or just claim to receive or do something. Most people use the words "right" and "entitlement" interchangeably, assuming both are free (no payment) and that everyone gets their right or entitlement whenever they want regardless of income, location, age, and for health care regardless of whether they are citizens or not.

ERISA = Employee Retirement Income Security Act of 1974. Creates standards for employer-sponsored health insurance plans, especially those who are self-funded. Many large organizations, from large hospitals to Walmart and Amazon, are self-funded for health insurance. ERISA rules supersede any state-level insurance rules.

Error/mistake (contrast to adverse impact) = an incorrect action or behavior. To make an error requires that the correct action or behavior is known and possible. So, in healthcare, if there is no medical choice that is proven to be "correct," then there cannot be a mistake, even if a patient has an adverse impact. (See Adverse impact.)

Exemption (or waiver) = means that an organization, group, or even municipality does not have to comply with the legal requirements of PPAHCA. Certain religious groups and more than 1,400 organizations—unions or businesses—have been granted exemptions.

FFM = Federally Facilitated Marketplace. This is the federally run program, created by PPAHCA, in which American citizens can and must purchase health insurance. The website's URL is www.healthcare.gov.

FPL = federal poverty level is a measure of income determined each year by the Department of Health and Human Services. FPL is used as a base line to define eligibility for Medicaid and CHIP amongst other federal social programs. In 2017, the FPL for a family of four was $28,290. With ACA setting Medicaid eligibility up to 138 percent of FPL, a family qualified with income less than $39, 040.

Fiduciary = a relationship between two people where person "A" gives control over himself or herself to person "B" so "B" can use this power for the benefit of person "A."

GAO = Government Accounting Office. Where the Congressional Budget Office (CBO) is concerned with the future, the GAO, also called the "Congressional watchdog," looks at the past. This agency assesses federal spending. For instance, in 1990 on the twenty-fifth anniversary of the Medicare Act, the GAO calculated how much was actually spent in contrast to how much the CBO budgeted or predicted in 1965. Congress and the CBO underestimated the cost of Medicare by 854 percent. (See CBO.)

Gobeille *v.* Liberty Mutual: See SCOTUS.

Guaranteed issue = rule that requires insurance carriers to accept any patient for coverage, regardless of any pre-existing health condition the patient might have and, thus, regardless of how much that individual might cost the insurance plan.

"Healthcare is a sick patient." = This is my way of saying that only a medical approach can fix our dysfunctional healthcare system. Political and financial approaches over the past 50 years have made the patient called "Healthcare" sicker, not healthier.

Health Insurance Exchange (HIE) = a major component of PPAHCA where people can shop for health insurance and those who qualify, which is 70 percent of the U.S. population, can obtain subsidies to reduce out-of-pocket costs. Eighteen states are operating their own exchanges. The majority has decided not to create state-based exchanges: their citizens must obtain insurance through the FFM at www.healthcare. gov. (See FFM.)

High-risk pool = refers to those Americans with expensive, usually chronic medical conditions whose annual medical expenses make it difficult-to-impossible to obtain health insurance.

HIPAA = **H**ealth **I**nsurance **P**ortability and **A**ccountability **A**ct of 1996. Intended to solve the problem of losing health insurance when losing a job—it did nothing to fix this. HIPAA created a massive regulatory machine, a host of burdensome rules, and tens of billions in costs, all supposedly to protect the confidentiality of medical information—and it doesn't.

HITECH = **H**ealth **I**nformation **T**echnology for **E**conomic and **C**linical **H**ealth Act. This was part of The American Recovery and Reinvestment Act of 2009. It was intended to create medical information technology standards and infrastructure, and to strengthen the security of personal health information.

Hobby Lobby decision = See SCOTUS: Burwell *v.* Hobby Lobby.

HSA = **H**ealth **S**avings **A**ccount. A bank account owned by an individual in which contributions are not subject to federal taxes. The funds can roll over through the years and accumulate. They can be used only for approved medical expenses. Obamacare limits the amount you can withdraw from an HSA.

ICD-10 = **I**nternational **C**lassification of **D**iseases. A complex, almost incomprehensible billing and coding system that doctors, pharmacists, therapists, and hospitals are required to use if they want to be paid. In addition to illness and injuries, ICD codebooks also include procedures, devices, and anything else that has to do with paying for health care goods and services.

IHS = Indian Health Service is a federal agency within the Department of Health and Human Services to provide health services to approximately 2.2 million American Indians and Alaska Natives. IHS is not an entitlement (enrollees pay); is not an insurance plan (it contracts with numerous insurers); and does not have a mandated benefits package like the ACA.

Incentive = is a motivator that either encourages someone to perform some behavior (colloquially called a "carrot" or reward) or discourages someone from doing something (a "stick" or punishment). Low prices, say, for insurance are a positive incentive to purchase. PPAHCA's tax penalty for not buying insurance is a negative incentive or "stick."

Individual mandate = refers to the cornerstone of PPAHCA: a federal mandate or requirement that each citizen (does not apply to non-citizens or undocumented immigrants) purchase health insurance. This was struck down by the Supreme Court, which then said it would be constitutional if it were called a "tax." It is the first time American citizens can be "taxed" (penalized) if they *don't* buy something, in this case, health insurance.

Insurance principle = where small contributions of the many pay the great (large) expenses of the few. Lots of people put small amounts of money into a common "risk pool," and a small number of people take out large amounts of money.

IPAB = Independent Payment Advisory Board. Created by ACA, this federal agency is tasked with reducing health care spending. It is imperative that you read more about this secretive committee, as it will directly impact what care you can receive and what may be denied to you. IPAB was recently renamed HTAC (Health Technology Assessment Committee). IPAB was what former Governor Sarah Palin famously called a "Death Panel" in 2009. Read more about this in *"The Cancer in the American Healthcare System."*

"It just stands to reason." = a phrase used by those who have no hard evidence to support their position or plan. They rely on appeal to emotion.

Job lock = being stuck in a job you do not want to do because you will lose your insurance benefits if you leave. In February, 2014 the CBO released a report predicting that PPAHCA would cause the loss of more than two million jobs in the U.S. Nancy Pelosi (D-CA, 12th District), a strong proponent of the ACA and former majority leader of the House of Representatives, hailed this result saying that Americans would no longer "be job locked but can [as a result of PPAHCA] follow their passion," meaning they could work at what they choose, or decide not to work at all.

King v. Burwell: See SCOTUS.

Learn = to acquire data, knowledge, understanding and (hopefully) wisdom. To learn requires you to question what you have been taught is true, and sometimes unlearn that so you can learn what IS true. As I have written, "Today's 'best medical practice' can be tomorrow's malpractice."

Little Sisters of the Poor v. Burwell: See SCOTUS: Zubrik v. Burwell.

MACRA = <u>M</u>edicare <u>A</u>ccess and <u>C</u>HIP <u>R</u>eauthorization <u>A</u>ct of 2015 changed how doctors are paid by the two named federal programs.

Market failure = market here means a "free market," where consumers spend their own money and where prices can vary. Market failure means that the free market does not allocate goods and services *efficiently*, giving the best and cheapest stuff to the most people. The usual alternative suggested to a free market is central (government) control, which has been shown over and over to be *inefficient*—giving the most to a small number of elite people and little-to-nothing to the public at large. This is not conservative bias. It is based on the hard evidence of history.

Medicaid = (contrast to Medicare) This is an *entitlement* program, in contrast to Medicare. You qualify by low income, age, or having certain chronic conditions. You pay nothing and receive benefits dictated by the government.

Medical malpractice (tort) system = When a patient is injured or harmed in relation to medical care, the malpractice system supposedly punishes the wrongdoer and compensates the injured. An alternative system called Office of Medical Injuries is proposed in Book 7, *We Don't Need Tort Reform . . . We Need Replacement.*

Medicare (contrast to Medicaid) = Medicare is *not* an entitlement program. You paid into it during your whole working career. Medicare was conceived as a giant Health Savings Account (HSA), where you put in money for 40 years. When you retire, that very large pot of money, which accumulated and grew, would pay all the medical expenses of your golden years. Read in *The Cancer in the American Healthcare System* how and why Congress subverted Medicare.

MERP = **M**edicaid **E**state **R**ecovery **P**rogram. Passed as part of the Omnibus Budget Recovery Act of 1993, this law allows state governments to recoup a $611-per-month administrative fee (which could total as much as $73,310) and property after the death of a Medicaid recipient. To this, the states can add a bill for 10–40 percent of a patient's total medical bills that were paid through Medicaid.

Metal level = Insurance plans that are ACA-compliant have different amounts (percents) of your health care costs that are covered by the Plan. Using the names of metals signifies these different levels: Bronze (60 percent of your costs are covered); Silver (70 percent); Gold (80 percent); and Platinum (90 percent). Of course, the cost of the insurance premium goes up considerably depending on which "metal" level you choose: Bronze = cheapest; Platinum = most costly. As the cost rises, the benefits also increase.

Micro-economic disconnection = refers to the separation of the consumer from control of his or her own money. This makes it impossible for the free market to function, as supply and demand can no longer balance each other.

Moral hazard = refers to the danger to society of some people spending other people's money and therefore having no need to economize or to act responsibly or morally.

Navigator = PPAHCA requires each state to have people available to help individuals through the complexity of purchasing health insurance. These individuals are presumably impartial, or not paid by or beholden to any insurance carrier, as brokers can be. Navigators are also called "in-person assisters."

Net (when calculating pretty much anything) = I frequently use this word because too many people look exclusively at the short-term cost, without considering long-term costs and without evaluating benefits at all. A "net calculation" for spending on healthcare would determine **value**—what we *really* care about—by comparing long-term costs and risks to long-term benefits to patients.

NFIB *v.* Sebelius: See SCOTUS.

NHS = National Health Service. This is the name of the government-run healthcare system in Great Britain. It was used as a model for the original version of Obamacare.

N.I.C.E. = <u>N</u>ational <u>I</u>nstitute for <u>C</u>linical <u>E</u>xcellence. A component of the NHS that was the model for the IPAB that is part of Obamacare. Both NICE and IPAB are tasked with cost cutting by deciding what medical care will be authorized and therefore available for use in patients. These groups also decide what types of care will be denied, or deemed Not Cost Effective, even if the treatment works medically.

Payer = can be confusing. In most aspects of your life, the payer IS the **consumer**; they are one and the same. In a free market, the consumer/payer gives money to the supplier in exchange for goods and services. Healthcare, with its third-party payer system, is not a free market. The consumer does not directly pay the supplier and therefore is not the payer. The **supplier** (provider) does not set his/her price. The government, not the market, determines the price. There is a third-party **payer** who either has no incentive to economize (the government) or is rewarded, or incentivized, when it denies payment for care (insurance).

PBM = <u>P</u>harmacy <u>B</u>enefits <u>M</u>anager. This is a computer program implemented by many health plans that doctors must use to order medications. The program tells the doctor what drugs he or she can or cannot use (usually determined by cost, not medical efficacy for that patient). If the doctor wants to use a non-approved drug, there is a complex, time-consuming process to appeal the health plan's restriction.

PCIP = <u>P</u>re-Existing <u>C</u>ondition <u>I</u>nsurance <u>P</u>rogram. A component of the Affordable Care Act that was supposed to provide insurance for those usually *uninsurable* because of expensive pre-existing medical conditions. Enrollment was discontinued after less than a third of the eligible people signed up. The chairman of the New Mexico High Risk Insurance Pool said, "Washington just left the sickest of Americans high and dry, holding nothing but an empty promise."

Perverse incentive = means that someone is rewarded when they do the opposite of what is wanted. In retail, this would be giving a bonus to the person who sells the least products. In healthcare, it is perverse when insurance makes profits by delaying, deferring, or denying medical care—the Strategy of the Three D's in Chapter 3 of Book 1—even though you need the care now!

Phantom code = a billing code used by a health care provider to charge for a service he or she did not actually provide. This is fraud.

PNHP = Physicians for a National Health Program. A political activist group that advocates for a single payer approach for the United States. Their position is discussed in *Single Payer Won't Save Us.*

Population medicine = doing what is medically best, as decided by some panel of experts (self-styled), for the population as a whole. That means the needs of the group supersede the needs of the individual. Doctors are ethically committed to the opposite: *personal* medicine.

Primum non nocere = Latin phrase considered the *prime directive* for physicians and is commonly but incorrectly translated as "First (above all), do no harm." A more precise interpretation of the original Latin yields, "At least, do no harm!"

Provider (of health care) = anyone whose activities *directly* affect a patient, such as a doctor, nurse, respiratory therapist, social worker, etc. Many others, not called providers, *indirectly* affect patient welfare, such as billers, coders, managers, legislators, regulators, support staff, technicians, etc.

Psychic reward = an emotional or psychological, non-material payment for a service, product, or action. For most health care providers, the psychic reward for helping others is more important than the monetary reward.

Public option = is a shorthand colloquial term for single payer, in contrast to having multiple entities, usually insurance carriers, but sometimes health organizations, who pay the costs for health care goods and services. Many use the Canadian system as an example of a public option.

Ration = to "make reasonable," or to apply logic and reason to a problem. In Economics, to *ration* is "to balance supply and demand."

Regulatory burden = a mountain of federal regulations that control every aspect of healthcare, from the financing to the day-to-day practice of medicine. The cost of compliance with these regulations is massive in money, in provider frustration, in medical errors, and time taken away from patient care *by federal mandate*. The dollar cost of the federal regulatory bureaucracy is now more than 40 percent of <u>all</u> U.S. healthcare spending.

Rent-seeking behavior = where a private company seeks to obtain economic advantage through government intervention such as tariff protection or cost-sharing reductions ("bailouts"). By definition, the economic gain does not produce any benefit to society through wealth creation. Rent-seeking is government redistribution to benefit a favored commercial enterprise.

Rescission = insurance industry jargon for canceling an insurance policy, sometimes for frivolous reasons or with a trumped-up excuse.

Right (to health care) = means you are entitled to health care (the service), when you want, where you want, what you want, for free, without needing to qualify in any way. Proponents say that by simply being alive, you have this right. The relationship between a right to health care and one's personal responsibility has never been openly discussed. I believe the lack of consensus on this matter is at the heart of problems in our healthcare system.

Romneycare = colloquial term for the Massachusetts health care insurance reform act signed into law in April 2006 while Mitt Romney was governor. The proper name for this system is Commonwealth Care. There are many similarities between Romneycare and Obamacare, but they are not identical.

Root cause ("etiology" is the medical term) = refers to the primary or first cause. This is the "why" of illness. In diabetes, the symptoms are related to elevated sugar in the blood, but elevated sugar is not the root cause, which is due to failure of insulin to regulate blood sugar. Dysfunction or improper production of insulin is the root cause in diabetes. Has anyone shown to you what the root causes are to explain why our healthcare system is "broken"?

SCOTUS = <u>S</u>upreme <u>C</u>ourt <u>of</u> <u>t</u>he <u>U</u>nited <u>S</u>tates. The five major ACA-related cases that have been heard by the Supreme Court are listed below:

1.   **2012: *NFIB v. Sebelius*** = The National Federation of Independent Business sued then-Secretary of Health and Human Services, Kathleen Sebelius, challenging both the individual mandate and the mandatory expansion of all state Medicaid programs. SCOTUS struck both down as unconstitutional. Then, in this 5–4 decision, they said the federal government could keep the individual mandate if they changed the name to a "tax." Medicaid expansion remained voluntary.

2. **2014:** *Burwell v. Hobby Lobby* = Obamacare requires all insurance to provide 10 essential benefits, which include contraceptives and abortifacients. Christian-based Hobby Lobby Company sued claiming that the ACA violated their right to religious freedom (First Amendment). After years of lower-court hearings, the Supreme Court heard the case, agreed with Hobby Lobby, and prohibited the federal government from penalizing religious-based organizations for failure to offer contraceptives and abortifacients.

3. **2015:** *King v. Burwell* = David King and three other plaintiffs sued Sylvia Burwell as Secretary of Health and Human Services. They claimed that the federal government was illegally providing subsidies because healthcare.gov is an exchange created by the *federal* government, but the ACA says subsidies can only be provided through exchanges "established by the *state*." The IRS issued a ruling that healthcare.gov could provide subsidies even though the ACA said it could not. In a 6–3 decision, SCOTUS upheld the IRS, opining they understood that Congress wanted to give subsidies to everyone, even if the law wasn't written that way.

4. **2016:** *Gobeille v. Liberty Mutual* = Vermont wanted to create a statewide database for healthcare. When they sought to require carriers to provide their information, Liberty Mutual refused, claiming federal law—ERISA, which is the Employee Retirement Income Security Act of 1974—prevented them from complying. The Supreme Court decided in Liberty Mutual's favor that federal

law superseded state law. The decision will reduce the amount of data available to consumers of care services.

5. **2016:** *Zubrik v. Burwell* = The Hobby Lobby decision (above) was written with very narrow applicability. Therefore, Obamacare was still allowed to use healthcare dollars to support, albeit indirectly, abortion, contraception, and "birth preventative services." A number of Catholic organizations led by the Little Sisters of the Poor sued the federal government claiming Obamacare violated their right to religious freedom (First Amendment). During oral arguments in April 2016, the justices took the unusual step of asking the litigants if they could settle their differences without a Court decision. The Little Sisters said yes, but the government said no. The Supreme Court then decided ... not to decide. Their unanimous, unsigned *decision* was to refer the case back to lower courts to find a compromise without holding either for plaintiff or defendant.

SHOP = <u>S</u>mall Business <u>H</u>ealth <u>O</u>ptions <u>P</u>rogram. This is a part of the ACA that offers insurance plans to small businesses.

Signup (enrollee) = Washington counts anyone who has completed the application process for insurance, even if that person is not covered, no card is issued, and/or the person has never paid a premium.

Single Payer system = where the government is the distribution source for payments to providers, institutions, suppliers, and (if insurance is used), insurance middlemen. Because it controls both the money and the regulations, the government dictates how much it will pay, what it will pay for, and when. There are no market forces in a Single Payer system such as those in a free market. Instead, a monopoly (government) controls both supply and demand. The U.S. Veterans Administration is a Single Payer system, as is the British National Health Service. (See Public option.)

Spending (noun) = money paid. All too often, "spending" is mistakenly used to mean the same as "cost," which is very different. (See Cost.)

Subsidy from ACA. See APTC.

System = a set of connected things or parts that form a complex structure. The key is the word "connected," because without the structure and minus the connections, parts are just a pile of stuff that can do nothing.

Systems thinking = a management approach that emphasizes the need to study the intact system or entire structure as a whole. When you break it up and study each part separately, you lose the connections and its "system-ness." Practicing good medicine on anyone requires systems thinking. A good doctor would never do something to improve kidney function without considering how that treatment might affect other organs such as the heart, lungs, or liver.

TANSTAAFL = "There Ain't No Such Thing As A Free Lunch." It means that nothing in this world is free, nothing. *Someone* has to pay for it, whatever "it" is.

The Three D's = a strategy used by health care payers to hold on to your money as long as possible: delay, defer, or deny.

"Trust me! I have your best interests at heart." = This is a common catchphrase of those who take a paternalistic attitude toward others and control them, for their own good, of course.

Two-master dilemma = the problem of who should be your first priority: your employer or your customer; your patient's best interests or following regulations. I call this the "who-master dilemma."

UMRA = Unfunded Mandates Reform Act of 1995. This act was intended to fix the problem created by EMTALA, which created the unfunded mandate: the law that requires hospitals to treat patients for free, which in turn makes them overcharge paying patients to avoid bankruptcy. As you can see, UMRA did not resolve the unfunded mandate, which is now an even bigger problem than it was in 1995. (See EMTALA.)

Uncompensated care = medical care that a hospital must provide by law for which it receives no payment—the unfunded mandate. This was an unintended consequence of EMTALA (See EMTALA.)

*Under***insured** = The purpose of insurance is to prevent financial disaster in the event of an expensive medical catastrophe. As many as 84 million Americans have medical insurance where the coverage is too low to protect them from medical bankruptcy. These are the "*under*insured."

Unfunded mandate. See EMTALA and Uncompensated care.

*Un***insured** = those who have no medical insurance. Current estimates put this number at 45–50 million Americans, 24 percent of whom are not legal citizens. Because of EMTALA, sick patients can always get care whether they have insurance or not, and it is paid for by someone else—in most cases, the U.S. taxpayer.

Universal health care = national healthcare systems where reputedly everyone gets care. I write "reputedly" because these systems are not *universal* (non-citizens do not get free care). *Care may be denied* by government decree and often is. For example, there is Canada, where people sometimes cannot get the care they need when they need it.

Up-code = provider submits a billing code for a service the provider did not provide, which generates a higher charge than the service actually provided.

"We the Patients" = We the Patients emphasizes our commonality—every person is now a patient or eventually will be a patient. We the Patients includes Democrats and Republicans, rich and poor, all ages and stages, and American citizens as well as people here illegally. If you are alive in the U.S., you are part of We the Patients. We are all in "this" together, where "this" means life in the U.S.

Index

Review Requested:

If you loved this book, would you please provide
a review at Amazon.com?

CPSIA information can be obtained
at www.ICGtesting.com
Printed in the USA
FFHW012236250119
50287965-55329FF